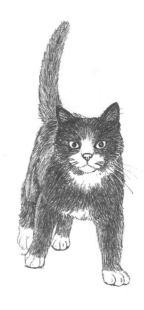

The
Veterinarians' Guide
to Your
Cat's Symptoms

Michael S. Garvey, D.V.M.

Ann E. Hohenhaus, D.V.M.

Katherine A. Houpt, V.M.D., Ph.D.

John E. Pinckney, D.V.M.

Melissa S. Wallace, D.V.M.

Elizabeth Randolph

VILLARD · NEW YORK

The
Veterinarians' Guide
to Your
Cat's Symptoms

Copyright © 1999 by Elizabeth Randolph and Lowenstein Associates, Inc.

Illustrations copyright © 1999 Rick Reason

All rights reserved under International and Pan-American Copyright Conventions. Published in the United States by Villard Books, a division of Random House, Inc., New York, and simultaneously in Canada by Random House of Canada Limited, Toronto.

Villard Books and colophon are registered trademarks of Random House, Inc.

Library of Congress Cataloging-in-Publication Data

The veterinarians' guide to your cat's symptoms / Michael S. Garvey . . . [et al.].
     p.   cm.
    Includes index.
    ISBN 0-375-75227-7
     1. Cats—Diseases—Diagnosis. 2. Symptoms in animals.
   I. Garvey, Michael S.
   SF985.V48 1999   636.8'089—dc21   98-39149

Random House website address: www.atrandom.com

Printed in the United States of America on acid-free paper

9 8 7 6 5 4 3 2

First Edition

DESIGNED BY BARBARA MARKS

This book is in no way meant to take the place of the medical advice of a veterinarian. A pet owner should consult a veterinarian regularly about the health of her or his cat, in particular if the animal shows any signs/symptoms of illness. The signs/symptoms listed in this book, and the medical conditions they may indicate, are in no way intended to be all-inclusive. They are merely the most commonly seen signs/symptoms in the clinical experiences of the contributing veterinarians.

For Higgins

and Misty.

May they continue

to live happy,

healthy lives.

Acknowledgments

Thanks to Mollie Doyle at Villard for her patience, calm, and understanding; and to Barbara Lowenstein, without whom this project would never have happened. Thanks in particular to Norman Kurz at Lowenstein Associates for his help.

Thanks also to Drs. Michael Garvey, Ann Hohenhaus, Katherine Houpt, and Melissa Wallace for their contributions, and especially to Dr. John Pinckney for his heroic efforts.

Last, but by no means least, thanks to my husband, Arthur Hettich, for his continuing encouragement and support.

—Elizabeth Randolph

Contents

Charts and Tables

Illustrations

A Note to the Reader

There are many books on the market designed to assist people in understanding their bodies and health. Several are based on symptoms of disease so that a person can find her symptoms and discover what the most common medical causes of these symptoms could be. There has not been a similar book for pet owners up until now. The authors have written this book to help pet owners recognize the medical causes of problems with their cats and take appropriate steps.

One of the difficulties in writing about medical topics for a nonmedical audience is terminology. Words have very specific meanings and are used very carefully in medicine. Many unfamiliar medical words will be used in this book and, because the intended audience for it is nonmedical, we have included a glossary of terms at the back of this book.

Among the terminology problems is the fact that the words *symptom* and *sign* are both used in this book. By definition, a *symptom* is a human patient's subjective observation of various pieces of evidence that something may be wrong, which she is able to communicate to her doctor. A *sign* is something that is objectively seen, felt, smelled, or heard. Because a cat cannot communicate her physical feelings except in the most general way (i.e., change in behavior), she technically cannot have symptoms and an owner or veterinarian must look for signs of medical trouble. However, because most people are familiar with the use of *symptoms* rather than *signs,* we have used both terms interchangeably in this book.

—Michael S. Garvey, D.V.M.

*The
Veterinarians' Guide
to Your
Cat's Symptoms*

Part One

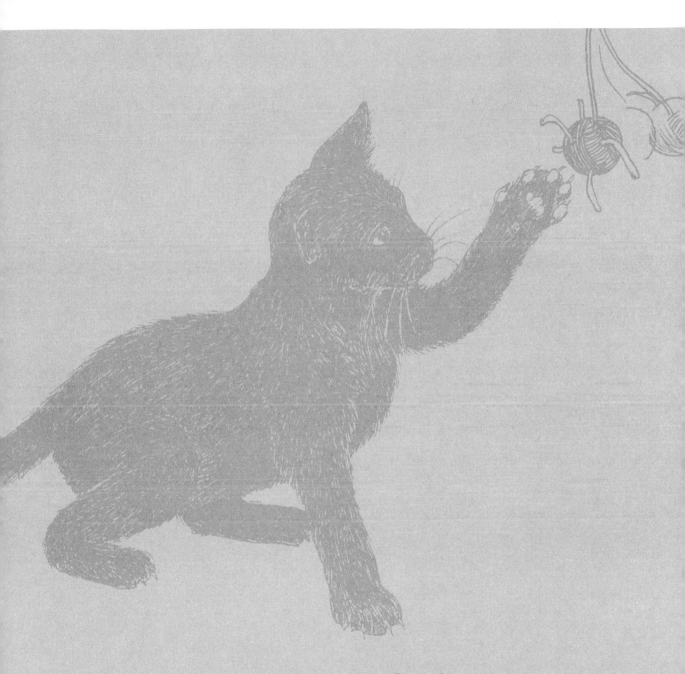

A Healthy Cat

A Healthy

Cat's Body

In this chapter is a short description of the various systems in normal, healthy cats' bodies, touching on the differences between cats and humans and among cat breeds. The primary purpose of this chapter is to provide cat owners with a basis of comparison in case a cat's body seems not to be functioning correctly.

In general, cats' bodies work in much the same way as those of all other mammals, humans included. However, cats are apt to develop different diseases and illnesses than other species do. These specific problems and diseases will be covered in the symptoms section of this book. Cats have also evolved over the ages to have particular abilities that meet their particular needs. For example, they have a very highly developed ability to see and "sense" in the dark; they are able to jump very high, turn their paws inward, and retract and extend their claws. We will learn more about these special skills in this chapter.

Although breeds of cats have been developed with a variety of body, face, and ear shapes, tail lengths, and hair coats, all cats are alike physiologically. There are, however, some differences among cat breeds. For example, manx cats, which are tailless, often suffer from congenital abnormalities of their hindquarters.

Skin and Hair

One of the most noticeable differences among cat breeds is the length of their hair, or coat. Cats' coats form an insulating layer between their skin and the external environment and protect them from the cold in winter and the sun in summer. Cats have three basic types of hair. Fine hairs make up a soft undercoat, while the outercoat is longer and coarser. There are also the stiff vibrissae, or whiskers, which project from a cat's body. These tactile, or sinus, hairs are unique to cats' bodies and include not only the whiskers but the eyelashes and sinus hairs on the insides of the middle forearms. Exceptions are rex cats, both Cornish and Devon. Cornish rex cats' coats have no guard hairs at all, and Devon rex cats have uneven coats and few whiskers. Both have short, curly coats that lie close to their bodies. Cats' whiskers are enervated by the fifth cranial nerve of the brain, and are able to act like radar, allowing cats to "feel" air currents and movements. Cats' hair can stand on end all over their bodies when they are afraid or angry because of tiny muscles that react in an action called piloerection.

All cats shed all year long. Outdoor cats shed more in the spring, as days begin to become longer. Different coat lengths and types of hair determine the amount of shedding, although all cats will shed excessively when they are under stress. It is especially important to groom long-haired cats regularly or the shed hairs will become matted and tangled instead of falling out.

Cats' skin plays many important roles. Not only does it protect a cat's body from loss of fluids, electrolytes, and proteins but it also serves as a barrier against infections. Cats do not perspire through their skin, but the skin does help maintain body temperature. The blood vessels in the skin either dilate to cool the body or constrict to retain body heat when it's cold. One of the skin's most important functions is as a sensory perceptor, conveying things like heat, cold, and pain to the brain.

A healthy cat's coat is shiny and full and her skin is clear and free of sores, scabs, redness, or scaly patches. If a cat is born with brown or black spots on her skin it is probably normal pigmentation, but if dark skin spots or discoloration suddenly occur they should be evaluated by a veterinarian.

Eyes and Vision

Although cats' eyes have essentially the same parts as humans and other mammals, they differ from all other animals' in several ways, enabling cats to have the best night vision of all domestic animals. Cats' eyes have a great many more rods than cones, while human eyes have more cones than rods. Because rods respond to very low light, cats can see extremely well in dim light. Also, their pupils are oblong instead of round, which enables them to dilate widely in low light, and thereby let in more light. In bright light cats' pupils become a very thin slit, protecting their eyes, which are sensitive to light.

Owners are sometimes concerned when a cat's eyes seem to have a bluish or yellowish glare if the animal is looking toward the light; blue-

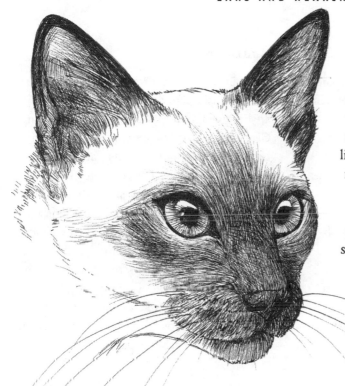

is a pinkish membrane that sometimes appears in the inside corner of a cat's eye, partially covering the eyeball. This membrane is called a third eyelid (nictitating membrane) and is present in all mammals except humans. The third eyelid pops up automatically when a cat retracts her eyes (pulls them back into the eye sockets). It protects and cleans the eyeball, and may become more noticeable if a cat's eye is irritated or if she is suffering from an illness. Burmese cats occasionally develop an eversion (outward turning) of the gland of the third eyelid, which can be surgically corrected.

Cats with prominent eyes and flat faces (brachycephalic breeds) such as Persians and Himalayans are more susceptible to eye damage because their eyes are not set deep in their sockets.

A typical example of a cat with a long, triangular head. Note the well-protected eyes and long, straight nose.

eyed cats' eyes will have a reddish glare. This is the reflection from a region around the retina called the tapetum. The tapetum reflects light back to the retina, further enhancing a cat's night vision. Older cats sometimes develop a condition called lenticular sclerosis, in which the lens fibers become dense and refract light differently, making the eyes look bluish. This condition does not affect a cat's vision but should be observed by a veterinarian to distinguish it from cataracts (see pages 110, 147, 148, and 149).

Another cause for possible owner concern

Ears and Hearing

Cats' internal ears have the same parts as humans'. All cats have pointed, upright ear flaps, or pinnae. Variations occur in Scottish Folds, whose ear tips are flipped forward, and American Curls, whose ears flip backward at the tips. Cats' upright ears help capture sounds and direct them down the ear canal to the eardrum, from where they are transmitted to the brain.

Cats' hearing is estimated to be at least three times more acute than humans' and they are able to hear high-pitched sounds much better than people. It is common for white cats with two blue eyes to suffer from congenital deafness.

Noses and a Sense of Smell

Cat noses come in variations of two basic shapes; pointed and flat-faced, or brachycephalic. Longhaired cats, such as Persians and Himalayans, have been bred to have extremely flat faces. Some shorthaired cat breeds such as British Shorthairs and Scottish Folds have somewhat flattened faces and protuberant eyes, but are not truly brachycephalic. Extremely brachycephalic cats may have upper respiratory problems due to their very small nasal openings (nares).

Cats' sense of smell is very acute because the olfactory (smell-sensing) areas of their brains are highly developed. Their appetite is mostly controlled by smell. Therefore, if a cat's nose is stuffed up, she will not be very interested in eating.

Mouth and Teeth

Cats' teeth serve two purposes. They are both offensive and defensive weapons, and also are designed to fit cats' particular style of eating. Cats grasp and then shred or tear their food before swallowing. Adult cats' canine teeth are slanted inward in order to trap prey better.

Kittens have twenty-six teeth, which are replaced by thirty adult teeth by the time a kitten is six months old. The teeth are evenly divided between the upper and lower jaws.

Cat tongues are very rough and serve primarily as grooming tools, smoothing fur and removing loose hair like a comb. If too much loose hair is swallowed, a cat will develop hair balls in the stomach (see page 140).

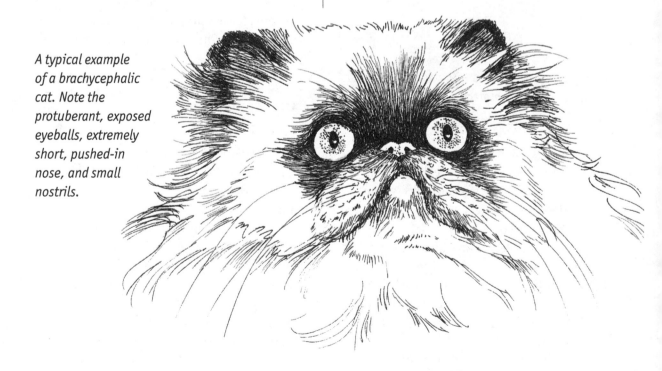

A typical example of a brachycephalic cat. Note the protuberant, exposed eyeballs, extremely short, pushed-in nose, and small nostrils.

Cardiovascular System

Cats' cardiovascular systems are similar to those of humans and other mammals. Cats have a four-chambered *heart* with two atria and two ventricles. A cat's heart is primarily responsible for pumping and circulating blood through an elaborate network of *arteries,* which deliver oxygenated blood to tissues, and *veins,* which drain deoxygenated blood from tissues and return it to the heart. It is then pumped into the lungs for reoxygenation during respiration.

In general, cats do not suffer from the types of cardiovascular disease that humans do. For example, arteriosclerosis, or plaques on the inside of arteries caused by an excess of cholesterol, is virtually nonexistent in cats. Nor do they suffer from heart attacks brought on by clogged arteries. Cats do, however, have other types of heart problems, which we will discuss later.

Digestive System

The digestive system of the cat is made up of components that transport food and fluids into and through the body. On the way through the digestive system, nutrients and fluid are absorbed and utilized by the body tissues. The remaining waste products are eventually eliminated.

The mouth and teeth grab and grind food until it can be swallowed and passed via the *esophagus,* a long muscular tube running from the back of the throat, to the *stomach.* In the stomach, food is further ground and churned. Stomach acids and small amounts of enzymes begin the digestive process. The resulting gruel then moves into the *small intestine,* where *pancreatic enzymes, intestinal enzymes,* and *bile* (produced by the liver) break it down into absorbable components. Fluids and these nutrients are absorbed through the lining of the small intestines. Remaining nonabsorbed material, including wastes for excretion, then move into the *large intestine* or colon. Most fluid is removed from this waste, and firm stool is produced and excreted via the *rectum.*

The liver is the largest organ in a cat's body. It is responsible for a myriad of important functions. In addition to producing bile to aid digestion, it acts to metabolize and detoxify any drugs, chemicals, or poisons that enter a cat's body. It manufactures the major blood-clotting factors, and stores sugar to provide energy between meals.

Endocrine System

The *endocrine glands* are located throughout a cat's body. They manufacture and release *hormones* into the bloodstream, which then travel to other organs and attach themselves, causing necessary functions to occur.

Some of the endocrine glands that are important are the *thyroid glands,* which exert a major impact on a cat's metabolism and regulate how rapidly the body's metabolic functions occur. The *parathyroid glands* are located near the thyroid glands and are important in regulating levels of calcium and phosphorous in the animal's bloodstream. *Adrenal glands,* which are near the kidneys, secrete a variety of important hormones, such as cortisol and others that regulate blood pressure and electrolyte balance.

Part of the endocrine system also includes a network of cells in the *pancreas* that secretes insulin and other hormones that help utilize and assimilate sugars and other nutrients.

There are also a variety of *reproductive hormones* that a cat's glands secrete. These are responsible for normal heat cycles, egg production, and uterine health in female cats, and normal sperm production in males.

If a particular endocrine organ oversecretes or undersecretes hormones, diseases occur in a cat's body, which will be discussed later in this book.

Musculoskeletal System

Like humans, cats have clavicles (collarbones), which dogs do not. Cats have a more flexible skeletal system than dogs do. A cat can compress her body, or "coil," allowing her to spring high from a standing or crouching position.

Cats have specialized muscles in their forearms that enable them to turn their front paws inward (pronate them) so they can bat or grasp prey or toys.

Nervous System

Just as in humans, cats' nervous systems are basically broken up into two different areas, the *central nervous system* and the *peripheral nervous system*. The central nervous system includes the *brain* and the *spinal cord*, which runs from the back of the brain through small bones or vertebrae in the spine along almost the entire length of a cat's body.

The brain is responsible for thinking, memory, cognitive function, and many other things. The spinal cord accepts impulses from nerves located everywhere on a cat's body, especially the legs and feet, and brings important information

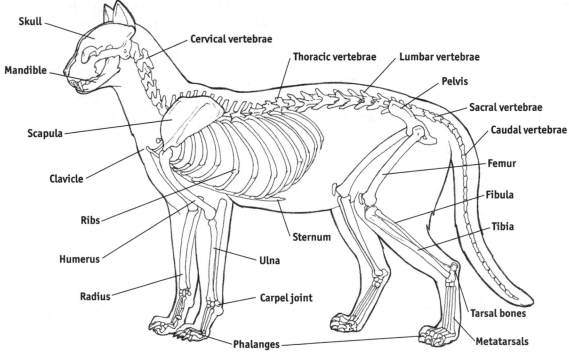

A Normal Cat's Skeleton

from peripheral nerves to the brain such as sensations of cold, heat, pain, and touch. It also transmits conscious and unconscious commands to the periphery of the body.

The *peripheral nervous system* includes the twelve cranial nerves that come out of the brain and are responsible for all of the things that occur from the neck up, including vision, smell, and hearing. Peripheral nerves branch out of the brain and the spinal cord also transmit messages to the muscles, telling them either to expand or contract so the cat can stand, walk, jump, and move normally. There is also a sensory component of peripheral nerves that relays sensations up the spinal cord.

Reproductive System

Cats' reproductive systems have the same components as those of all other mammals.

The age when a female cat enters puberty depends on when she was born and can vary from five to twelve months of age. This is because cats are what is called seasonally polyestrus, that is, their estrus (heat) cycle depends on the amount of daylight (photoperiod) in a day. In the Northern Hemisphere most cats begin to cycle in February or March and continue to cycle every two to three weeks until fall, unless a cat is mated and becomes pregnant. Approximately twelve to fourteen hours of light a day is the normal measure used. Persian cats are the exception; they enter puberty as late as one and a half years of age. Indoor cats that live in nothing but bright artificial light, on the other hand, may cycle all year long. Signs of estrus in female cats are mostly behavioral. Cats in estrus will become very affectionate, vocalize a lot, become agitated, and walk with their backs arched and tails extended. They

also roll around on the floor; this behavior can be so dramatic owners may confuse it with seizures.

Female cats have a total of eight *mammary glands,* four on each side of the body. In young cats these glands are not very prominent and look like little specks. In older females, particularly those who have had a litter of nursing kittens, the breasts may be more prominent and pendulous. In older, unspayed female cats the mammary glands may develop tumors. Cat breast tumors, while less common than in dogs, are often highly malignant. If an owner detects a lump in the area of the mammary glands, a veterinarian should be consulted immediately.

Surgical neutering prevents many health problems in both male and female cats and protects females from unwanted pregnancies. Unneutered male (tom) cats usually spray foul-smelling urine markers all around their territories, which makes them most unpleasant house pets. For the greatest health benefits females should be spayed (have an overiohysterectomy) before their first heat, at anywhere between six and seven months of age; males should be castrated by the time they're eight months old so that spraying urine doesn't become a habit. In recent years many shelters have found that both male and female kittens can be neutered at much earlier ages with no ill side effects. This earlier neutering has been effective in preventing unwanted kittens. For more about this, see "Spaying and Neutering" in the following chapter, page 20.

Respiratory System

A cat's respiratory system brings oxygen into her body to be carried into the bloodstream, and eliminates carbon dioxide (the waste product of organ metabolism) from her body. The respiratory system starts with the *nose* or *mouth,* which brings air to the *trachea,* or windpipe, a long hollow tube that begins at the back of the throat. Air is brought through the trachea to the *lungs* through a branching network of smaller tubes called *bronchi* and *bronchioles.* The lungs are an elaborate network of membranes with very small blood vessels through which oxygen can pass and enter the bloodstream. Anything that interrupts this process of oxygenation, such as lung or bronchial disease, will cause difficulties because a cat's body will not get its required oxygen supply. Cats who exhibit difficulty breathing should be handled very carefully. Any stress can cause hypoxia (low blood oxygen), which causes cats to become wild and uncontrollable and often leads to death.

Urinary System

The urinary system of all mammals, including cats, is primarily responsible for maintaining body water balance, i.e., assuring that the body has the proper amount of water at all times. The *kidneys* regulate this by removing water from urine before it is excreted, or by allowing water to be passed in urine when it is excreted. Two very long, thin tubes, called *ureters,* connect the kidneys to the *bladder.* The bladder is a hollow, muscular organ that stores urine and then contracts to excrete it. Kidneys also provide an important function in removing toxins and waste products from a cat's body.

Unlike all other mammals, male cats do not have a discrete large *prostate gland.* Instead, they have several very small, scattered prostate glands. Therefore, they are able to avoid the prostate gland problems many other species often have.

Other Systems

Paws and claws: Cats usually have five toes on each front foot, and four on each back foot, but they sometimes have extra toes on their front feet and occasionally on their hind feet. This is an inherited trait called polydactyly.

Cat footpads are thick and smooth. Sweat glands are located between their footpads.

Cats are able to extend and retract their claws by using specialized muscles, tendons, and ligaments. Cat claws serve several purposes. They are used as weapons, as an aid in climbing, for catching prey, and for digging to bury waste. If a cat's claws do not wear down naturally, they must be clipped to prevent them from catching on things and damaging people and other pets.

Anal glands: Cats have anal glands, or sacs, on either side of the rectum that contain a foul-smelling secretion. The secreted matter in the anal glands is forced out when a cat defecates. Unlike dogs, cats rarely suffer from impacted anal glands, but anal gland abscesses have been seen occasionally in cats.

How to Keep
a Cat's Body
Healthy

Just as is true in human health care, the best way to assure a cat's physical well-being is to practice common sense care and preventive medicine. Proper veterinary care, immunizations against contagious diseases, nutrition that meets a cat's needs at each stage of his life, basic grooming and cleanliness, some kind of play or exercise, and generally good daily care all combine to form a routine that will help a cat's body function at its maximum potential.

Choosing a Veterinarian

Before bringing a new kitten or cat home, it's a good idea to shop for a veterinarian, because a thorough head-to-tail checkup is one of the very first steps to take in sensible preventive medicine.

Although there are low-cost clinics that will perform most routine services such as yearly immunizations and boosters and simple neutering operations, most cat owners want a veterinarian with whom they can consult if some aspect of their pet's well-being troubles them. For this purpose a good companion animal practitioner is the best choice, especially for pet owners with both cats and dogs. As a good pediatrician does with a child and his parents, it is important that a veterinarian get to know both pet and owner in order to be effective in assessing illnesses and disorders that may arise later on in a cat's life. There are veterinarians who limit their practices to feline medicine only, but they are not necessarily feline specialists. Cats-only veterinary practices may be more satisfactory for owners of particularly timid cats, which may not appreciate an office full of barking dogs.

Veterinarians differ greatly in ability and personality, just as human doctors do. For general, routine pet care, probably the most important aspect in selecting a veterinarian is an owner's ability to get along with and communicate well with the doctor. In case something very complicated should come up, a general-practice veterinarian will usually refer a pet owner to a specialist in the area of concern, such as dermatology, cardiology, internal medicine, and so forth. It's a good idea to find out ahead of time if the veterinary practice being considered has access to these types of specialists, or to a large veterinary teaching facility or hospital with specialists on staff.

The best sources of information about local veterinarians are pet-owning friends and neighbors. Breeders, groomers, and even pet-supply-store owners may also know of good local veterinarians. Many veterinarians are in group practice and share facilities and staff. Barring any of these resources, call the American Animal Hospital Association (AAHA) toll free (see page 165 for the number). They have the names of member animal hospitals in all geographical areas. They set high standards for their animal hospital members in equipment, procedures, and physical facilities.

Nowadays a great many animal hospitals are closed on Sundays, holidays, and during nighttime hours. For off-hour and holiday emergencies several practices often join to establish a centrally located emergency clinic, manned by member veterinarians and employees on a rotating basis. If this arrangement is not satisfactory it may be best to find a veterinary practice in which one of the doctors is on call all of the time.

Once a preliminary decision is made to choose a particular veterinarian and/or practice, an appointment should be made for a checkup for a new kitten or cat as soon as possible after he comes home. At that time, if an owner finds the veterinarian is not satisfactory, common sense dictates that another doctor be found. More about what to expect on the first veterinary visit later in this chapter.

Choosing a Healthy Pet

The first decision a potential kitten or cat owner has to make is, purebred or mixed breed? There are advantages to each kind of cat, and a lot depends on an owner's lifestyle and the expected lifestyle of the pet.

If a potential owner has decided on a particular kind of cat, a purebred may be ideal. Purebred cats differ from mixed-breed cats in that they have been selectively bred to develop particular body conformations, haircoats, temperaments, and personalities. It's important for a potential owner to be aware of the differences among breeds. Persian cats are quite different from Siamese, for instance, just as British Short-hairs are very unlike Abyssinians. A purebred kitten raised in good conditions by a reliable breeder will grow into an adult cat with a predictable haircoat, body conformation, and so on. Some cat breeds may be prone to particular physical disorders. For a list of some congenital diseases and defects common to particular breeds, see Appendix B, page 147.

For first-time cat owners who know they want a purebred cat, the best source for a kitten is a breeder. It is very unusual to find an adult purebred cat for sale. Breeders and owners of purebreds are generally very devoted to their cats and will not part with them. Unlike the American Kennel Club for dogs, there is no one, central registry of standards for purebred cats in the United States. One of the best ways to locate a breeder is to visit one or more cat shows: talk to breeders and cat owners and see the kittens and cats. For someone who wants a pet, not a show cat, breeders will often offer what they call a "pet quality" kitten with less-than-show-perfect markings for a price less than that for a show-quality kitten. Purebred-cat breeders are usually very careful of their animals and take good care of them, although there are exceptions. Even the most careful breeder may not be able to prevent all disease, so it is still very important to visit a veterinarian immediately.

Breeders often travel far to attend cat shows so it may not be possible to see the parents or littermates of a kitten being considered. If a purebred kitten has been raised in a private home, on the other hand, a potential owner should be sure to see both parents to make certain a kitten actually *is* purebred and not the product of accidental mating, and to evaluate their health and personalities. It's important for a kitten obtained from

any source to visit a veterinarian right away, and for a new owner to obtain a binding return agreement should the kitten turn out to have a serious defect or disease.

Serious cat breeders are very unlikely to sell their pets to chain pet stores. The kittens in these stores are generally obtained from opportunistic breeders who want to cash in on the popularity of certain cat breeds and who may have little interest in proper genetics or preventive health care.

Nearly 90 percent of pet cats owned in this country are mixed breeds. Mixed-breed cats are generally healthy and hardy and make excellent pets. Mixed-breed kittens are not difficult to find, especially in the spring when the breeding season is at its height. Kittens, and grown cats, too, of all combinations of colors and haircoats can be located through Humane Societies, shelters, or even advertisements on supermarket bulletin boards. For first-time pet owners, and owners who want a special cat, the best bet is to find a kitten or cat that has been raised in a caring home in which the mother of the kittens is someone's well-loved pet. A kitten from this kind of home will have been born into a relatively clean, disease-free environment to a mother who has been well fed and is probably parasite free.

However, little kittens are especially vulnerable to disease, and even loving pet owners may not be aware of the necessity to immunize them. Be sure to obtain a vaccination and health certificate signed by a veterinarian if you opt to adopt a kitten from a private home. Then take the new kitten or cat to the veterinarian right away to have a complete physical examination, and additional immunizations if necessary.

If there are other cats in the household, isolate the newcomer until he's given a completely clean bill of health. A minimum of two weeks is recommended to be certain a new pet isn't incubating an infectious disease that even a veterinarian may not be able to detect (see *incubation periods,* below). This means providing separate living quarters, litter pans, food and water dishes, and toys. Even if the existing resident cats have up-to-date immunizations, there may be strains of disease to which they are not immune. This is especially true in the case of very young or elderly cats, who are apt to be less resistant to disease than healthy young adults.

If a new kitten or cat is obviously unwell, or develops symptoms of illness, even stricter care is necessary to protect resident felines from exposure. An owner can become a carrier of viral diseases on clothing, shoes, and hands. Protective clothing, such as a smock and gloves and old socks and slippers, should be worn over regular clothing when taking care of a sick newcomer, and this clothing should stay in the "isolation room." Careful hand washing after handling a sick cat is a must. If these steps seem difficult, remember, it is much easier to prevent infection than to have several sick cats to take care of.

A Veterinary Checkup

Many young kittens have roundworms. Left unchecked, roundworms can cause a kitten to have diarrhea and eventually become very sick. They can also infect humans. Roundworm eggs are shed in the feces of an infected kitten, and if they are ingested by a human can migrate to various organs, most particularly the eyes, where they will eventually cause blindness. Since most young children frequently put their unwashed hands into their mouths, this is especially important to know if there are young children in the household. Roundworm eggs are not infectious when first passed. They need time to become contagious, so frequent emptying of litter pans is very important. Because of the serious nature of roundworm infections in humans it is essential that a kitten be dewormed, even if no worms are visible in a stool sample. Treatment with proper medication should be given at least twice at two-to-four-week intervals, usually at the same time immunizations are given. The medication is safe, effective, and not expensive. Over-the-counter products are usually unsatisfactory and can be dangerous for a small kitten.

The veterinarian will check the kitten all over, from head to tail. She'll listen to his heart and lungs, check the insides of his mouth and ears for any abnormalities or signs of ear mites, and feel his rib cage and stomach for any swelling or abnormality. She'll check the kitten's skin and coat. She'll check the kitten's genitals and determine his (her) gender. She'll weigh the kitten in order to keep a record of growth, and take his temperature. She will also perform blood tests to be sure the kitten is free from either the feline leukemia virus (FeLV; see page 161) or feline immunodeficiency virus (FIV; see page 161), both of which are retroviruses and lead to serious illness.

If a kitten or cat seems to be in general good health, the next step is to establish an immunization schedule. Kittens need to be vaccinated against infectious diseases every few weeks in order to be fully protected (see page 18). If a kitten is going to be an indoors-outdoors pet, ask the veterinarian at what stage in the immunization process it will be safe to allow him outdoors. Owners should be aware, however, that indoor-only cats are much healthier than those that are allowed out, and tend to live longer.

No matter if a cat is strictly an indoor pet, he still needs protection from dangerous infectious diseases. He can be exposed to disease organisms from infectious feces brought in on peoples' shoes, by viruses that are airborne, or carried on clothing and hands, by insect carriers, and by exposure to other pets in veterinary hospitals. Immunity to disease is not a lifetime condition for cats but must be reinforced regularly for the animal to remain protected. Adult cats need revaccinations, called booster shots, to retain immunity from disease. They are usually given every year, except rabies. See page 19 for an adult cat's booster schedule.

One piece of equipment that should be mentioned here is a sturdy carrying case for a cat. The cardboard boxes that are often given to new cat owners are not really escapeproof. A roomy, hard-sided case with a latched door is a good choice (see illustration, page 49). Soft-sided, nylon-mesh cat carriers are also popular. Most veterinarians insist that cat patients come to their offices in carrying cases.

How Do Vaccinations Work, and What Do They Prevent?

Vaccinations help a cat's body develop *antibodies,* which fight off specific infectious diseases by awakening his body's immune system to the particular bacterium or virus that causes the disease when it invades the animal's body. An antibody is a protein that is manufactured in the cat's body when it is exposed to the disease organism in the vaccine. Vaccines are used to prevent diseases, not treat them, and will do no good if a kitten or cat is already infected with a disease.

The infectious cat diseases for which vaccines have been developed are: feline panleukopenia, rhinotracheitis, calicivirus (these three are often prevented with one vaccine); pneumonitis, also called chlamydia (which may be included in four-component vaccines); feline leukemia virus (FeLV), and rabies (killed vaccine only for cats). Veterinarians usually recommend the three-component vaccine because pneumonitis is relatively mild and uncommon in household cats. If a cat is boarded or taken to cat shows, pneumonitis vaccine is often added. Upper respiratory infections such as rhinotracheitis and calicivirus can be very serious in cats and may lead to death.

A vaccine to prevent feline infectious peritonitis (FIP) is now available through veterinarians. The vaccine is different from the injectable ones mentioned above. It is given in a cat's nose, because the nose is where the FIP virus is thought to enter the cat's body and cause infection. The remainder of a cat's body is warmer than the nasal passages and this increased temperature causes the virus to die so it cannot infect the entire cat. Not all veterinarians feel this vaccine is necessary or effective because kittens are usually affected with FIP shortly after birth. Indoor-only cats are not at risk for acquiring FIP because it is caught from other cats. The need for this vaccine should be discussed with a veterinarian.

One of the things for owners to remember is that various diseases have different *incubation periods,* or lapses of time between exposure to the disease and the actual outbreak of the disease. During the incubation period of a disease an animal will show no signs of illness; it isn't until the disease has spread throughout a cat's body that he will become visibly ill. This lack of symptoms is especially common with young kittens that have not been given good health care. It is very important to begin a kitten's immunization process right away; the so-called temporary shots often given to kittens are not very effective—see below for more details about this. If a kitten is started on an immunization schedule while he is incubating a disease, it is really a matter of chance whether the disease or the antibodies will win. Sometimes seemingly healthy kittens that are in the process of being immunized can sicken and even die because of this.

Chart 1:
RECOMMENDED VACCINATIONS FOR ALL KITTENS

(Note: The vaccines contained in shots given to kittens may vary according to individual veterinarians. These are the vaccinations we believe all kittens should have.)

Disease	6–8 wks.*	9–12 wks.	13–15 wks.	16+ wks.
Panleukopenia/ Rhinotracheitis/ Calicivirus (PRC)**	+	+	+	
Rabies			+	

*Not all veterinarians begin vaccinations this early.

**PRC immunizations for kittens should be given every 2–4 weeks from the time they are started until the kitten reaches the appropriate age.

Chart 2:
OTHER VACCINATIONS THAT ARE AVAILABLE FOR KITTENS

These vaccinations are not routinely given to all cats, especially indoor-only cats. A veterinarian may recommend them if he feels they are indicated.

Disease	6–8 wks.	9–12 wks.	13–15 wks.	16+ wks.
Feline leukemia virus (FeLV)*		+	+	
Feline infectious peritonitis (FIP), given nasally				+
Pneumonitis**		+	+	

*A blood test is performed first to be sure the infection is not present.

**Required by some boarding kennels.

There is currently a controversy about feline immunizations. A growing number of people believe cats are being vaccinated too frequently and do not need yearly boosters. Opponents are afraid that if the frequency of vaccinations is reduced, the result will be the return of many feline diseases. At the time of this writing, we still recommend following the schedules found here.

It is very rare for a vaccination to cause a cat to become ill, but beginning in 1991 several reports in veterinary medical journals associated the administration of feline vaccines with the development of skin tumors (sarcomas) at the spot where the vaccine was given. This occurred most often when killed rabies vaccines and FeLV vaccines were given. The current thinking is that a chemical called an *adjuvant,* added to these two vaccines to stimulate the immune response, is responsible for the tumor development. An adjuvant is *not* present in other cat vaccines. The incidence of these tumors is low—approximately one in five to ten thousand vaccinations. In the future, vaccines will be produced with advanced DNA technology that may help eliminate the risk of cats developing these tumors.

Vaccinations are usually given in a series every four weeks to kittens under four months of age. See the kitten immunization chart, on page

Chart 3: RECOMMENDED VACCINATIONS FOR ALL ADULT CATS		
Disease	**Yearly**	**Every 1–3 years depending on type of vaccine used**
Panleukopenia/ Rhinotracheitis/ Calicivirus (PRC)	+	
Rabies		+
Note: PRC should be given one year after the last kitten immunization. The first rabies vaccination is good for only one year, no matter what type of vaccine is used.		

Chart 4: OPTIONAL VACCINATIONS FOR ADULT CATS
The following vaccinations are available for cats and should be given to cats that go outdoors or associate with many strange cats, at the veterinarian's discretion.
Feline leukemia virus (FeLV), given only after a blood test to be sure the disease is not present
Feline infectious peritonitis (FIP), given nasally
Pneumonitis—may be required by a boarding kennel

18. This is necessary because the *passive immunity* kittens attain during the first week of life from the colostrum in their mothers' milk is short-lived. Studies show that 95 percent of kittens have lost passive immunity by the time they are twelve weeks old; most of the remaining 5 percent lose it by the time they are fourteen weeks old. While the maternal antibodies are present they automatically inactivate a vaccine. But because we don't know exactly when this passive immunity will be lost, a series of vaccines is given to ensure a kitten's immunity at all times. After fourteen weeks it is almost certain a kitten no longer has any maternal antibodies and he will now be able to respond to vaccination by forming his own antibodies, or *active immunity*. This is why so-called temporary shots do not always provide effective protection.

After a kitten has been successfully vaccinated by the series of injections it can usually be assumed that immunity has been achieved for a period of time. But owners must realize no vaccine is 100 percent effective in all cases. Some cats have a more sluggish immune system than others, and not all respond as well to vaccines as others. It is always possible for a kitten or cat to contract a disease even when he has been properly vaccinated, although the disease will usually be less severe and of shorter duration than it would be in an unprotected animal. Booster shots are given to adult cats on a regular basis (see page 19).

Spaying and Neutering

At the same time the veterinarian sets up an immunization schedule she will probably want to discuss the benefits of spaying or neutering a pet cat.

If an owner does not want to breed a pet cat, both an overiohysterectomy (OHE, "spay") of a female cat and castration ("neutering," "altering") of a tomcat are desirable for a number of reasons both behavioral and physical. In both cases, of course, these operations prevent accidental breeding and the birth of unwanted litters of kittens. Although public awareness has reduced the number of unwanted kittens in recent years, a visit to any pound or shelter, especially in the spring and early summer breeding season, will attest to the continuing birth of many hundreds of unwanted kittens each year. Many of these kittens are not adopted and end up being put to sleep.

In addition to preventing the conception and birth of kittens, an OHE will also prevent recurring heat periods in female cats. During heat periods female cats will pace and yowl, or "call," loudly all day and night. They will usually also rub continuously against both people and furniture and may roll around on the floor. Because cats normally do not ovulate unless they are bred, heat periods will continue to occur every ten to fourteen days during the entire photoperiod (see page 11). When a female cat is spayed before her first heat period, the operation is thought to prevent mammary gland tumors, which are very serious in cats, and will also prevent future uterine infections and tumors of the reproductive tract.

Although an OHE is a major abdominal operation, modern medical techniques have made it relatively painless and uncomplicated when performed by a competent veterinarian. A cat will usually stay in the hospital overnight following an OHE to be certain she has come out of the anesthetic well and is comfortable. After a day or so of quiet rest at home she usually shows no signs of discomfort. Complications rarely occur, but if a cat should show signs of discomfort or the incision becomes red or irritated, the veterinarian should be consulted.

For a male cat castration usually eliminates roaming behavior, aggression toward other cats, and, probably the most important consideration for a pet owner, the spraying of foul-smelling urine to mark his territory. Once a cat forms this habit it can be very difficult to break, so castration before eight months of age is recommended. Neutering also decreases the odor of male cat urine.

The neutering operation is relatively simple and a cat is usually allowed to go home the same day. After the operation the cat needs to be kept indoors for several days to prevent infection. Shredded newspaper should be substituted for clay litter to prevent contamination of the incision. Complications are rare; the most common problem is swelling of the scrotum due to irritation or excessive licking. If this occurs the veterinarian should be consulted.

In recent years many animal shelters have begun to neuter young kittens before they are adopted in order to avoid the birth of more unwanted kittens. So far, early neutering has proved to be safe and effective. However, not enough time has elapsed since this procedure was begun to find out if there are any negative long-term health effects. If a kitten from a shelter has already been castrated or had an OHE, there is probably nothing for a prospective owner to worry about. If the procedure has not already been performed, it is best to wait for the operations until the recommended ages.

What About Weight Gain After Spaying or Neutering?

Because OHE's and castrations are routinely performed just as cats are maturing, normal changes in sleeping habits, activity levels, metabolic rate, and food utilization are often blamed by owners on the surgery. However, some cats seem to have increased appetites after neutering. Owners need to remember that a one-year-old cat requires far fewer calories a day than a growing kitten.

Adult cats often need to be encouraged to exercise to burn off excess calories. Indoor-only cats, especially, may require incentives to exercise. More about this later in the chapter.

Providing Good Nutrition

Much has been learned about cats' nutritional needs in the past decade. Although cats' dietary requirements are similar to those of other mammals, it is known that they have some very specific and unique nutritional needs.

First of all, cats require more *protein* per day than dogs and this protein must come from an animal source in order to contain the amino acids necessary for cats. The amino acids *arginine* and *taurine* are essential for cats to have in their daily diets. Arginine helps rid adult cats' bodies of the unusually large amount of ammonia created by their high-protein diet. Their bodies cannot make arginine, therefore it must be part of their daily food. Arginine deficiency can lead to depression, muscle tremors, lack of coordination, and eventually death. Deficiencies are not common because meat proteins contain arginine. Taurine is not sufficiently manufactured in cats' bodies either, as it is in all other species. It is necessary that taurine be in a cat's diet throughout his lifetime. A deficiency of taurine will lead to degeneration of the retina and eventual blindness. It will also lead to severe, potentially life-threatening weakening of the heart muscle and stunted growth. Meat is the best source of this amino acid. Commercial pet food manufacturers are aware of cats' taurine requirement and add it to their products in the proper amount. Cats consuming home-cooked diets or vegetarian diets may be at risk for taurine deficiency.

There are three essential fatty acids that cats need: linoleic, linolenic, and arachidonic acid. Linoleic and linolenic acid are found in vegetable oils, but arachidonic acid is contained *only* in animal fats. An animal source of *fats* is essential for cats because, unlike other animals, cats cannot convert arachidonic acid from linoleic and linolenic acids.

Other essential dietary elements for cats include *vitamin A* and *niacin*. Cats have a relatively high vitamin A requirement, but are unable to convert carotenoids (found in vegetables) into vitamin A in their own bodies and must have a meat source for it. Liver is a good source for A, but an excess of liver can lead to severe bone disease caused by too much vitamin A. A deficiency of A can lead to weight loss, scaly skin, hair loss, and retinal and reproductive problems. Another essential dietary element that cats cannot convert in their own bodies is niacin, therefore they must have it in their daily diets. A niacin deficiency can lead to weakness, weight loss, diarrhea, mouth disorders (including a susceptibility to herpes), and respiratory disease.

Given the very specific dietary needs of cats, it is obvious that the best source of proper feline nutrition is a diet that has been formulated to meet these daily requirements. It is very difficult to meet these needs with a diet consisting only of home-cooked foods. Some owners opt to use a commercial cat food as a basic diet, adding home-cooked treats from time to time. Care must be taken, however, because some cats cannot digest even the blandest "people food," and will develop diarrhea. See also "Foods to Avoid," page 26.

To avoid upsets a new kitten or cat should be fed whatever type of food he has been used to eating. Breeders often send home a "care package" with several days' supply of food to start a kitten off on the right paw. If it becomes necessary or desirable to change diets, it's best to do so gradually, mixing a small amount of new food with the old. If a cat accepts the mix well, without any intestinal upset, increase the new food gradually each day until he is eating the diet exclusively.

Kinds of Cat Food

Commercial cat foods come in three basic forms: dry, semi-moist, and canned. The most obvious difference in these types of food is moisture content, which also affects their ability to stay fresh when exposed to air. Many owners feed their cats more than one type of food each day. It is a good idea to accustom a cat to eating several types and flavors of food early in life to avoid firmly established food preferences—see "Finicky Eaters," below. The most important thing about choosing cat food is that the label says "complete and balanced." Then any form of food is fine for a cat. Many owners feed a combination of dry and canned foods.

Vegetarian diets will not provide a cat with enough usable protein, taurine, essential fatty acids, and minerals to maintain health. Cats often like vegetables, and some vegetable matter is contained in almost all commercial cat foods. Cats are able to utilize carbohydrates and fats for energy, but they have an obligatory need for energy from protein sources even when they are fed enough other calories.

Semi-moist foods, once popular, are falling out of favor. While some cats loved them, the chemical odor was not appreciated by others. Many semi-moist foods are preserved with a high sugar content and many contained propylene glycol, which can damage cats' red blood cells. We do not recommend semi-moist diets, although an occasional semi-moist treat is all right.

Special-formula (prescription) diets are designed to meet the specific needs of cats with medical conditions such as food-related allergies, feline lower urinary tract disease (FLUTD; see page 54), heart condition, kidney failure, and so on. Their formulas are precise and they can be obtained only by prescription through veterinarians. Most are available in both dry and canned forms.

Finicky Eaters

Some cats are more particular about their food than others. In general there are several kinds of finicky eating. The most common type is when a cat develops a preference for one particular type or flavor of food, usually some sort of fish or chicken. If fish is preferred, it won't hurt a cat as long as the food is properly formulated and balanced. Problems can arise if a cat develops a preference for plain, unsupplemented fish intended for humans. Some fish contain an enzyme that breaks down thiamine, an essential vitamin. Another problem with all-fish diets is steatitis, a serious disease causing inflammation of body fat. This won't hurt a cat as long as the fish is properly supplemented and balanced (see chart, page 25).

Cats with chronic nasal congestion or those with a diminished sense of smell, which can occur in older animals, can also become problem eaters; as we mentioned in Chapter 1, cats' appetites are governed by their sense of smell. Upper respiratory infections can become chronic and prevent a cat from smelling his food and, therefore, from eating. Chronic nasal congestion can be treated by a veterinarian.

A cat may also reject food if he is upset for some reason. A move, a new pet or person in the household, a favorite animal or person going away—all of these events may cause a cat to lose his appetite. Other, more subtle changes may upset a cat, especially if he has a nervous temperament. Visitors in the household, sudden loud noises from outside such as building or street construction, a new feeding dish—anything can trigger a sensitive cat to lose his appetite. An owner will have to become a detective in this case to ascertain what may be upsetting a cat.

Sometimes there is no apparent cause for a sudden loss of appetite. If a cat is acting normal in other ways it is safe to wait a day or two, offer the cat's favorite food, and see what happens. Generally, a cat will begin to eat well again in a few days. If not, a veterinarian should be consulted right away.

How Much/How Often to Feed

Cats do not do well on one meal a day. Many owners leave dry food out all day for snacking and give one or two "meals" of canned food to their adult cats. Others do not like leaving food out and simply provide two larger meals a day. If food is left out all day some cats will overeat and become obese. See "Eating Behavior" in Chapter 3, pages 34–35, for more about this.

Avoiding Excessive Weight Gain

It is unusual for active indoor-outdoor cats to become overweight, but housebound pets may become obese because of inactivity. It is important for an obese cat to lose weight because excess weight puts a strain on a cat's body and will shorten his life. Obesity predisposes a cat to diabetes mellitus and will exacerbate respiratory conditions and arthritis.

A veterinarian is the best source of advice as to how to help a fat cat lose weight. A fat cat needs to have a lower caloric intake and usually can't be allowed to snack freely. Usually a veterinarian will prescribe a low-calorie cat food. The cat should be weighed regularly to be sure he is losing weight; otherwise his rations must be further reduced. Rapid weight loss in cats should be avoided, however. Some cats develop a poorly understood disease called hepatic lipidosis (fatty liver) from rapid weight loss.

The fatter a cat becomes, the less he is apt to move around. An owner can help a fat cat reduce his weight by encouraging him to play. A dangling object may entice him to play, or a small moving toy such as a ball (Ping-Pong balls are excellent) or a windup mouse may cause him to give chase. Don't expect a sedentary cat to suddenly jump up and play for any length of time. Give him a chance to get used to moving around again in short play sessions.

Feeding a Kitten

There are foods available on the market designed to meet kittens' special nutritional needs. Up until four months kittens should be fed four times a day; after that, at least twice a day. In general, kittens should be allowed to eat as much as they want at each feeding. Supplementation is not recommended as long as a kitten is fed a high-quality complete and balanced diet specifically for kittens.

Water

There is a common belief that cats don't require much drinking water because they can often obtain enough water from their food and seemingly drink very little. But, just like all living creatures, cats require water to replace fluids lost from waste, respiration, grooming, and evaporation. It is needed to flush out the body, to remove excess minerals and other waste materials, and to transport nutrients throughout a cat's body. If a cat loses body moisture due to a fever, diarrhea, or vomiting, he will need more water than usual.

A cat's water bowl should be kept clean and replenished daily. A bad-smelling water bowl or one with day-old film on top of the water will prevent a cat from drinking. Some cats prefer to drink water from a dripping faucet, shower stall floor, or even a toilet bowl. If a cat prefers water from fixtures, be sure to rinse off any cleans-

Kitten playing with a dangling toy.

Table 1:
DEFICIENCIES IN A CAT'S DIET: CAUSES AND RESULTS

Nutrient	Cause of Deficiency	Results
Arginine	Unsupplemented diet of foods high in casein (milk, cheese)	Depression, lack of coordination, muscle weakness, collapse
Taurine	Unsupplemented diet of dog food, vegetables, milk	Blindness, heart failure, stunting
Essential fatty acids (linoleic, linolenic, arachidonic)	Lack of dietary animal fat source	Low energy, poor coat, hair loss, sterility, crankiness
Vitamin A	Lack of animal tissue dietary source	Skin and eye problems, weight loss, impaired reproduction
Vitamin E	Diet high in unsaturated fats due to feeding unsupplemented dark, oily-meated fish	Pansteatitis, or yellow-fat disease
Vitamin K	Warfarin* poisoning, liver disease	Anemia, bleeding
Vitamin B$_1$ (Thiamine)	Diet of some kinds of raw or canned fish containing thiaminase; unsupplemented food that has been heated in processing	Anorexia, weight loss, convulsions, catatonia
Niacin	Lack of niacin in diet	Weakness, weight loss, mouth disorders, respiratory disorders
Biotin	Too many raw egg whites	Secretions around eyes, nose, mouth; emaciation, dermatitis
Calcium	Improper calcium-to-phosphorus ratio, unsupplemented all-meat diet	Soft, brittle bones; secondary hyperparathyroidism
Iron and copper	Unsupplemented all-milk diet	Anemia
Iodine	Unsupplemented all-meat diet	Thyroid dysfunction

*Warfarin and similar chemicals are components of rat poison.

	Table 2: EXCESSES IN A CAT'S DIET: CAUSES AND RESULTS	
Nutrient	**Cause of Excess**	**Results**
Vitamin A	Exclusive diet of raw liver	Severe bone disease
Vitamin D	Oversupplementation	Calcium and phosphorus deposits in soft tissues, renal failure, uroliths (urinary-tract stones)
Calcium		Soft-tissue mineralization
Magnesium	Too much in diet	Formation of uroliths
Vegetable matter	Too much in diet, unbalanced	Produces alkaline urine, which can lead to uroliths

ing materials. Other cats drink from standing water in plant saucers. This should be discouraged because chemicals may leach out into the water from soil and clay containers. If milk agrees with a cat and doesn't give him diarrhea, a small amount of milk each day is fine in addition to free-choice water. Special "milk" made for cats, which is more digestible than cows' milk, is available.

FOODS TO AVOID

Unlike dogs, cats usually won't eat potentially toxic "people food" such as chocolate. But a glance at the charts, above, shows that an excess of certain foods without proper supplementation—in other words, foods not designed specifically to meet cats' nutritional needs—can eventually lead to illness. The "bad" foods most commonly fed to cats in excess are unsupplemented fish (red tuna especially), raw liver or other meat, uncooked eggs, raw fish, dog food, and dairy products. Many cats cannot tolerate dairy products at all; milk in particular often gives adult cats diarrhea.

Indoors Only, or Outdoors-Indoors?

Although many suburban and country cats fare well going in and out of the house at will, unsupervised outdoor activity is very likely to shorten a cat's normal life span of fourteen to twenty years.

Even neutered cats are apt to stray from the safety of their yards and are susceptible to accidents and injuries. Fights with other cats can lead to cat-bite abscesses and exposure to infectious diseases such as feline leukemia virus and so forth. Cars, strange dogs, wildlife, unkind or thoughtless humans, and environmental dangers such as poisons used to kill weeds, insects, and rodents may also pose a danger to free-roaming cats. Cats that are allowed outdoors should always be called in at least twice a day for meals and to be sure they're all right. Many owners prefer to keep their indoor-outdoor cats inside at night for safety reasons. Cats that go outdoors, even if they rarely leave their yards, should always wear a collar and identification tag in case of a problem. An implantable microchip to identify a cat is another option. There are "breakaway" collars on the market that assure a cat can't become stuck or hung up on a branch—this used to be the reason many owners didn't put collars on their cats.

A cat owner who lives in a house or apartment with a balcony or terrace can provide a pet with the best of both worlds by securely screening an area where the cat can safely see the outdoors. A wide windowsill next to a screened window, or shelf attached to a

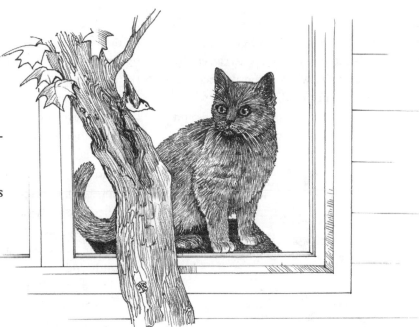

A window perch can provide an indoor-only cat with a safe and entertaining view of the outside world.

windowsill (available from many mail-order catalogs) is another alternative. An indoor cat can spend time very happily watching birds and squirrels from a windowsill perch. But the window must be screened; contrary to popular belief, a cat can easily fall or jump from a dangerous height, which will cause serious injury or death.

Some owners opt to teach a harnessed cat to walk on a leash. There are special figure-eight harnesses made for cats that allow them to move around safely and comfortably. The best time to teach a cat to wear a harness is when he is young. Starting off gradually indoors, a cat can become accustomed to the feel of the harness and eventually to the leash. Practice in the safety of a backyard or other quiet place will help a cat feel secure on a leash. He can then be taken for excursions on a regular basis. No matter how well a cat walks on a leash, it's a good idea to avoid noisy,

busy streets or areas where there are apt to be a number of other cats or loose dogs. Never leave a cat tied up alone in a yard where he cannot escape from a dog or wild animal.

Other Exercise/Play

We mentioned some games to play with cats in "Avoiding Excess Weight Gain," above. There are a number of different kinds of cat furniture on the market designed to encourage indoor activity—pet stores and pet supply catalogs are full of examples in all colors and styles. Although much of it is very attractive, it is also quite expensive and, unfortunately, doesn't necessarily appeal to all cats. Many owners prefer to make their own play furniture or provide a cat with recycled toys—a sturdy cardboard carton, an empty brown paper bag, a paper towel roll, or crinkled-up cellophane or tissue paper can pro-vide a lot of fun for a cat. Never give a cat string, ribbon, or thread to play with. Cats can easily swallow these items, which can make them very sick and may even be fatal. String items when swallowed are called linear foreign bodies and cause intestinal obstruction.

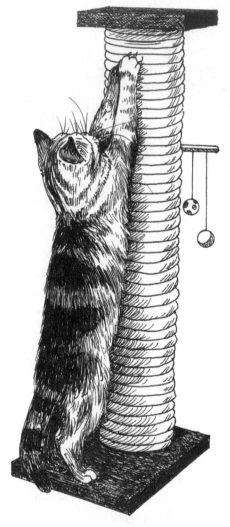

Cat using a scratching post. Note the sturdy base of the post, and the fact that it is tall enough for the cat to stretch out to her full length.

All cats with front claws, whether indoor-outdoor or strictly indoor, should have a suitable scratching device, not only to prevent damage to furniture and carpets but to provide good exer-cise and stretching for the cat. It may take an owner several tries to find just the right type of scratching post for a cat, but it's well worth the effort and expense. Scratching devices come with various coverings—carpet, sisal, or other sturdy fabric. Some cats prefer to scratch horizontally, others vertically; still others do both as long as the devices are covered with a favorite material. Be sure whatever scratching post is chosen is sturdy and heavy enough to be topple resistant, and long or tall enough for the cat to stretch out full length. Once the cat and scratching device have been matched, it is usually not too difficult to teach a cat to use the device for sharpening his claws, rather than the furniture. See Chapter 3 for more about this.

Grooming

One of the most important reasons for reg-ular brushing and combing is to remove loose hair. Because cats groom and lick themselves constantly, ungroomed cats swallow an enormous amount of hair, which will lead to the formation of hair balls (see page 140).

Regular grooming not only keeps a cat clean and free from snarls and mats, but it also does a great deal to keep his skin and coat healthy. A grooming session is an excellent time to look the animal over for wounds, sores, lumps, rashes, and parasites. A cat's ears should also be examined. Excess wax or dirt can be gently removed with a cotton swab, but be careful not to insert the swab any deeper than into the visible portion of the outer ear. A foul smell, black discharge, blood or pus are usually signs of an ear infection or infestation with ear mites (see page 108). A veterinarian should be consulted if there seems to be an ear problem. Most cats learn to enjoy being groomed as long as they have become accustomed to it gradually. The best time to introduce gentle grooming is when a kitten is young.

If a cat is skittish and afraid of grooming he may have had a bad experience. One way to help him get over his fear is to purchase a pair of grooming gloves, which are available in most pet-supply catalogs. These cotton gloves have small, soft bumps on the palms that act as a very gentle brush and remove some loose hair as the cat is stroked. Once a cat is used to being stroked with the gloves, a soft brush can be introduced.

Most owners find it convenient to assemble grooming tools in a bag, box, or drawer near the usual grooming location. Grooming is easiest to perform on a table or countertop. Shorthaired cats can be brushed to remove loose hair and then combed. If the air is very dry, a damp cloth rubbed over the surface of a shorthaired cat's coat after grooming will help collect any flying fur. Longhaired cats are easier to comb. If a long-haired cat is combed daily, most mats can be avoided. If mats do develop in a longhaired cat's undercoat, they should be pulled out gently, or cut out very carefully. It is very easy to cut a cat's skin when attempting to cut out mats—the best method is to cut a little bit into the center of the mat and then work it out gently. If a cat develops a lot of mats or the mats are very difficult to get out, he will have to be professionally shaved or clipped. Mats cannot be allowed to remain in a longhaired cat's fur; eventually they will cause sores, skin problems, or in severe cases, they can cut off circulation to a limb.

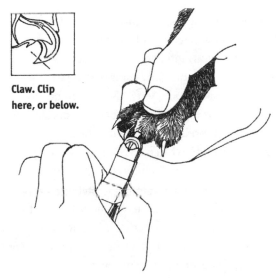

Claw. Clip here, or below.

Holding a cat's paw for claw clipping.

Cats' claws grow continuously and even outdoor cats who often scratch on rough bark or other material need to have their nails clipped regularly. Regular nail clipping prevents acciden-tal scratching of people or other animals and damage to furniture or rugs. Overlong claws can also catch on things, break, bleed, and may cause a cat to twist his leg or shoulder if a claw becomes caught in something.

Most cats learn to accept nail clipping calmly. Many owners prefer to sit with the cat on their lap, backside against their body. With one hand, grasp the cat's front paw. Press gently on the bottom of the cat's footpad to extend a claw and clip off the sharp, curved point with a claw clipper, being careful to avoid the nerve and blood vessel ("quick"), which are visible inside the claw at the thick base. If a cat is uncooperative and refuses to allow his feet to be held, it may be necessary to engage the help of another person to hold the cat. Some cats may become extremely upset and frightened when they have to be held as tightly as is necessary for claw clipping. Be careful that both people protect their arms and hands from scratches and/or bites, which can result in serious infection.

If an indoors-only cat is particularly intractable about allowing his claws to be clipped, or is especially destructive, a declawing operation is preferable to giving the cat away. Declawing is also often advised for households in which there are small children or disabled individuals, to prevent accidental scratching. Only the front claws are routinely removed, except in extreme cases. Although the operation is fairly routine nowadays, it is definitely not pleasant for the cat, and is best performed at a young age, often at the same time as a spaying or neutering operation.

An alternative to declawing is to surgically cut the tendons controlling the claws. This prevents a cat from extending his claws and damaging rugs, people, and furniture. The claws are not removed and must still be clipped on a routine basis. However, this procedure makes it easier for a cat to catch his claws in fabric. There is also a nonsurgical alternative using commercially available vinyl nail covers, or caps, which are glued over a cat's front nails to prevent scratching. Owners can learn to attach these covers themselves. These are an acceptable alternative to declawing for some, but the nails continue to grow and the caps often fall off.

Bathing a Cat

Although cats are usually not bathed, they *can* be bathed if needed. Sometimes circumstances such as a severe flea infestation, an encounter with a skunk, a bad bout of diarrhea, or contamination of the cat's fur by something poisonous makes it necessary to bathe a cat.

If an owner opts to bathe a cat herself, it is highly recommended that she have a helper hold the cat while she bathes him. Care must be taken not to chill a cat, and the room in which the bath is given should be warm and draft free. The best place to bathe a cat is in a waist-high tub or kitchen sink—a double sink is ideal, one for washing and the other for rinsing. Cats are often frightened by the sound of running water so it is best to fill both sinks with warm water ahead of time. Ample towels, shampoo diluted in warm water, and a washcloth to sponge the cat with should be nearby.

Before beginning the bath, protect the cat's eyes with a drop of mineral oil in each, or use an eye lubricant provided by a veterinarian. Lamb's wool, which doesn't absorb water, can be placed in his ears to protect them. If this is not available, cotton balls will do.

Very little shampoo is needed; too much will be hard to rinse out. It is very important to rinse all of the shampoo out to prevent skin irritation. Wrap the cat in a towel, pat him dry, and comb through his fur gently. Keep the cat in a warm, draft-free room until he is thoroughly dry.

If this process seems too difficult, or there is no helper available, most dog-grooming establishments, and some veterinarians, will bathe cats.

Fleas and Ticks

Ticks rarely become attached to cats because cats groom themselves so assiduously. But they may become attached to the edges of a cat's eyelids and other ungroomed areas. However, cats are especially susceptible to fleas, which can often be detected when grooming a cat, especially if a flea comb is used. Fleas can usually be found on cats in the thick fur on the back of their necks, on the spine at the base of the tail, and in the warm armpits and between the hind legs.

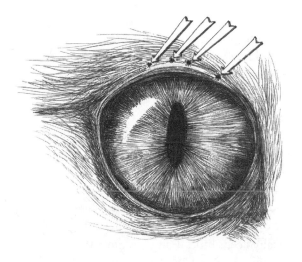

Although ticks usually do not adhere to cats, they may sometimes be found along the margin of a cat's eyelid.

Sometimes the fleas themselves can be seen. They are tiny, dark brown insects that jump very high and fast. Usually what owners see is flea "dirt," in the form of tiny, comma-shaped black specks.

If a cat is badly infested with fleas it may be necessary to give him a bath (see above) or to use flea powder, spray, or foam designed *especially* for cats. The veterinarian will be able to advise an owner about what kind of flea product to use and how to use it. If a flea infestation is not heavy, combing the cat thoroughly with a flea comb several times a day will trap fleas and flea eggs in the comb's teeth and remove them.

There are now excellent products on the market that are taken internally, or placed on a cat's fur, once a month during flea season (all year long in warm climates). They either repel or kill fleas or interfere with their reproductive cycle.

However, it isn't enough to repel fleas or kill the fleas on a cat because these parasites do not *live* on cats, but simply *feed* on them. There-

fore, environmental control is extremely important. Even an indoor cat in an indoor environment can become infested—dogs that go outside, for instance, can bring in fleas. In order to control a flea population it is necessary to rid the entire environment, outside and in, of fleas. There are a number of different ways to do this. A veterinarian, groomer, or other professional will be able to help determine the best method to use in a particular climate or environment.

Tooth Care

Veterinarians recommend regular tooth care for all cats to prevent tooth and gum problems when they get older. Without proper care a cat's teeth will develop tartar and invisible plaque, which inevitably will lead to inflammation of the gums (gingivitis), and tooth loss.

There are toothbrushes and toothpaste made especially for cats available from veterinarians and pet specialty stores. Human toothpaste shouldn't be used. Cats do not like the foaming or the taste, and it can cause stomach irritation. If cat toothpaste is not available, use a mixture of baking soda and salt, slightly moistened with water. A small, soft, child's toothbrush can be used instead of one made for cats. A finger "brush" made of soft rubber with small bumps projecting from the surface also works well.

Before undergoing a tooth-cleaning routine, an adult cat who has never had proper tooth care should have his teeth cleaned by a veterinarian to remove tartar that has built up over the years. Just as with all grooming routines, the earlier a kitten becomes used to having his teeth cleaned, the easier it will be. Begin by using a rough cloth wrapped around a finger and rub the teeth from gum to tip. Work up to a rougher cloth and then a toothbrush. This should be done approximately once a week unless the veterinarian recommends more frequent cleaning.

If there are signs of gingivitis (inflamed gums that bleed easily), broken teeth, or any swelling or redness inside a cat's mouth, he should be checked by a veterinarian.

Litter Trays

Even if a cat is allowed outdoors, at least one litter tray should be available to him in case of an emergency or very bad weather.

If there is more than one cat in a household, more than one litter tray is desirable. For two indoor cats, for instance, most owners keep two litter trays in different locations. (Note: Behaviorists often suggest that, to prevent problems, owners provide one more litter tray than the number of cats—for example, three litter trays for two cats.) Many cats won't use a litter tray that has been used by another animal, or one that isn't clean. Cats that are not well, or older cats, should have readily accessible litter trays. The location of a litter tray is important. Most cats like a little privacy when they use a litter tray. Once a suitable location has been found for the litter tray, it should not be moved if possible. If it has to be moved for some reason, be sure the cat knows where it is or he may be forced to use an inappropriate spot.

There are several different types of cat litter on the market. The principal kinds are clay and sandlike clumping litter. Cats often have definite preferences as to the type of litter they like. If possible it is best to stick to whatever type and brand of litter a cat is used to because cats are very conscious of texture and may reject a different kind. Clumping litter is very convenient and easy to clean but it is easily tracked around the house and has recently been reported to cause intestinal problems if it is ingested.

Litter trays, too, differ in style. Some cats prefer a covered litter tray while others are afraid to go in them. An owner will quickly find out if this is the case.

Solid waste should be removed from litter trays every day, and all of the litter should be changed on a regular basis. How often this is needed depends on the number of cats in a household, and the degree of fastidiousness of the cats. If plastic liners are used, the tray itself usually needs little, if any, cleaning. If they are not, the tray should be washed thoroughly. If disinfectant is used, care must be taken to rinse it off completely because any residual odor will offend a cat and force him to find alternative spots.

When an owner is observant of a cat's litter-tray preferences, many house-training problems can be avoided. See also "Elimination Behavior" in the following chapter.

Normal Cat

Behavior

Cats can be loving, affectionate companions. They are clean, soft, and small, are often cuddly, and are usually quiet and calm—a combination of traits that makes them especially ideal pets for older people and apartment dwellers. The fact that they do not need to be walked and are able to be left alone for fairly long periods of time without suffering from serious distress also makes them excellent pets for people who have to be away from home all day (although most pet cats greet their owners' return with signs of affection). An added plus for working people is that cats are crepuscular by nature, and one of their primary activity times is in the evening, when owners have returned home from work.

In this chapter we will describe normal cat behavior so a first-time owner will know what to expect. We will also cover several of the most prevalent types of inappropriate feline behaviors and provide some suggestions about how to deal with them.

Social Behavior

Are cats basically social animals or are they generally independent and aloof, as many people believe? There is great flexibility in the social system of cats. In the wild, cats are generally a nonsocial predatory species—that is, they are usually solitary hunters (with the exception of lions). However, when there is a concentration of food, which is always due to human activity, cats often live in large groups. But in a human household cats are more apt to be social and respond to people, other cats, dogs, and even other pets that might normally be considered prey, such as hamsters and birds.

A great deal depends on how a kitten has been raised. If she was gently handled by humans on a regular basis at an early age (the critical period is between two and seven weeks), she will usually respond positively to human handling as an adult. If this handling has not occurred, she is likely to be fearful of human contact and may never be able to be taught to be social with new people. It is also generally thought that a kitten raised with other kittens will become more socially responsive to other cats in a household when she matures, although some cats are loners by nature. By the same token, a kitten that has been raised with a friendly dog will be much less apt to be fearful of all dogs than one who has never encountered a dog before adulthood, or one who has had nothing but negative relationships with dogs.

At the usual time a kitten is adopted (around eight weeks of age), she is already housebroken and is quite mature physically. She is well coordinated and physically able to climb and jump, for instance, although she still has to grow to adult size and sexual maturity. She is already past her critical socialization period (the time during which she learns about her littermates, humans, and the environment), which means that it may take a while for an owner to establish new patterns of behavior in a kitten of this age.

Sleeping Behavior

Domestic cats sleep a great deal both during the day and at night. As a rule, they spend at least ten hours a day sleeping, interspersed with short bursts of activity. As we mentioned above, they are crepuscular and are most active at both dawn and dusk. Cats are often hungry in the early morning but don't want to eat by themselves and try to wake their owners by meowing or walking across them while they sleep. Owners who do not want to be awakened by a hungry or playful cat three hours before the alarm clock goes off find that if they leave a dish of dry food in the bedroom, it will at least temporarily satisfy and distract a cat.

Like all mammals, cats' sleep alternates between light or wakeful sleep (slow-wave sleep, or SWS) and deep (REM) sleep. Just like humans, dogs, and other mammals, cats dream during REM sleep.

Cats do not sleep in one spot all of the time, but change the "favorite" place where they sleep during the day from time to time (the exception is at night, when many cats sleep on their owner's beds). They will sleep in one chair for a few weeks, then switch to a bed, then the sofa, and so on. Behaviorists think this may be a form of instinctive parasite control.

Eating Behavior

In contrast to dogs, which usually eat during daylight hours, cats eat both night and day. A peculiarity of domestic cats, which they share with lions, is that they do not like sugar and water mixed, so will not lick sweet liquids, although they do not mind sugar and fat mixed and will often eat human desserts, for instance, given the chance.

Left to their own devices (free-choice feeding), cats will eat as many as twelve times a day. Owners are often troubled if a cat displays signs of being finicky and does not eat certain foods or doesn't eat much at all. A relatively little-known fact that may help explain this is that cats have been discovered to have innate cycles of body weight. If a cat is on one of the down cycles of her body weight, she will not have much appetite. If the cat is eating nothing, rush her to the veterinarian. As long as a cat is still eating something on a regular basis, and the period when a cat is "off her feed" does not last too long (more than a month or so), an owner should not be concerned; nor should he rush out and change cat foods, although it won't hurt. Cats particularly like novelty in their food and welcome a change of flavor, for instance. This is perfectly all right if the diet is complete and balanced for cats, and as long as the formulation of the diet is not changed drastically so as to upset a cat's digestive system.

Grooming Behavior

Cats groom themselves often and their grooming pattern is programmed. For instance, cats always wash their faces with their front paws exactly the same way, starting in small circles around the nose and then up around the ears. They then lick the rest of their bodies in order; some may end up cleaning between their footpads. Cats groom themselves after eating, upon awakening from a long sleep, and after being handled. If a cat suddenly stops grooming herself, it is a sign that something may be seriously wrong with her.

Cats in the same household also frequently groom each other. Mutual grooming can be arousing and may precede either sexual behavior or aggression. What begins as gentle grooming can become harder and harder and lead to a wrestling match.

Because of cats' continual grooming it is very important for an owner to keep a cat brushed and as free as possible from loose fur, which can be ingested and cause the formation of hair balls (for more about hair balls, see page 140). This is especially true in the case of long-haired cats, which are apt to groom themselves more frequently than shorthairs, but which also need owner help in order to keep their coats free from mats.

Territorial Behavior

Cats are territorial by nature. Males have larger territories than females in a natural situation, often encompassing females' territories. That is why it can be difficult to integrate a male cat, either castrated or not, into a household where there are other cats because he may try to drive all the other cats away.

Feline territories vary with the food supply. In a natural situation where cats have to hunt for food, each cat has her own territory. But when the food supply is concentrated, such as in a garbage dump, a granary where there are a lot of rats, or a fishery, for example, then many cats can live in the same area. In these situations each cat will have a small territory, or several cats may "time-share" a territory—that is, one cat may rest in a place from one to three o'clock, another from three to five, and so forth. Fortunately, unlike dogs, cats usually share food fairly amicably, although many do not get along with others in a home situation because of their territorial nature. Two cats get along much more readily than three or more in the same household. It can be very difficult to predict problems in a multiple-cat household.

Unneutered male cats (tomcats) mark their territories with foul-smelling urine. In fact, they produce a sulfurous-containing substance found only in cat urine (felinine). Neutered males and females, spayed or not, often mark also. See below, page 39, for more about this.

Cats also mark by scratching and with scent glands located in their cheeks and the upper surface of their tails. They will wind their tails around objects or people, or bunt (cheek rub) them.

Clawing Behavior

All cats claw regularly for several reasons. The first reason is to stretch; another is to get rid of loose claw material; the most important reason a cat will claw is to mark her territory. Clawing can be a social behavior, too. A good example of this is when an owner comes home and a cat immediately goes to the nearest prominent object and claws it. Outdoors, a cat will scratch on the trees that are in the area she frequents most—this is not to mark her territory but is a more social aspect of clawing.

We discuss suitable scratching devices for cats in Chapter 2, pages 27–28. It is helpful to have several scratching devices in a household, each placed in front of whatever piece of furniture is most prominent in the room, and another next to a favorite resting place.

Spraying urine against an upright object is a form of marking behavior used mostly by intact (unneutered) males. It may also be used by neutered males and some female cats.

Feline Communication

Cats use body language and facial expressions to communicate with other cats and with humans. For example, a cat that is greeting a person or another cat will hold her tail high, raised up in the air. One that is frightened will crouch, ears flattened to head, and she will salivate and spit. See below for a chart of some of the most common feline postures and facial expressions.

Vocalization

Cats make a number of different sounds that they use to communicate with other cats and with humans. They meow in greeting and to demand attention from their owners; growl and hiss in fear and anger; and caterwaul—the latter is usually a cat-to-cat communication between fighting tomcats. There is a similar call a cat gives when carrying prey. It is also like the sound a cat will make before vomiting up a hair ball. Adult cats do not usually purr when alone, but they do

Table 3: FELINE BODY LANGUAGE					
	Body	**Tail**	**Ears**	**Eyes**	**Vocalization**
Dominance Aggression	Standing on tiptoe, head slightly down, rear end higher than front	Curved downward, possibly fluffed slightly	Perked and swiveled backward	Constricted or half-dilated pupils	Growling, caterwauling
Fear	Crouched; paws close together; salivating	Wound around body	Flattened to head	Pupils dilated	Spitting, hissing
Fearful Aggression	Standing up straight, feet close together, back humped, mouth open	Hair on end	Flattened	Pupils fully dilated	Spitting, hissing
Greeting/ Investigating	Upright	High, straight up	Perked forward	Wide open	Meow, mew, murmur, squeak
Hunting/ Stalking	Low, close to the ground	Low, tip wagging	Pointed forward	Wide open	Very low growl; chattering, especially if unable to reach prey

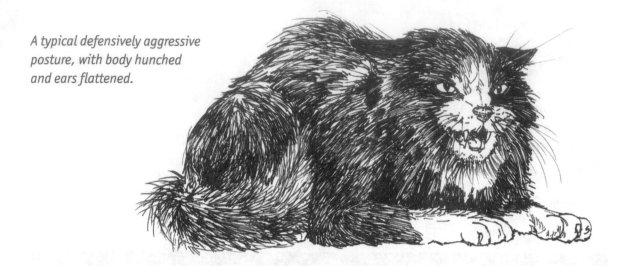

A typical defensively aggressive posture, with body hunched and ears flattened.

purr as a means of communicating with an owner, just as kittens purr to their mothers.

The sounds owners hear most frequently from pet cats are meowing and murmuring. There are breed differences in cat "voices." Siamese and Abyssinians, for instance, have very loud, raucous, and insistent meows, while Persians' meows are softer. Some owners encourage their cats to meow, or meow back to them, on signal. The demanding meow signifying "let me out," "feed me," and so forth is easily recognized. Behaviorists don't know exactly why some cats meow to their owners for no apparent reason.

Communicating with a Cat

Owners communicate with their pet cats by talking to them, stroking them, grooming them, and patting them. Most cats prefer to be petted under the chin rather than on top of their heads. Some cats enjoy gentle stroking, others like harder, firmer petting. An owner has to discover what method suits his pet best. Cats can be very demanding when they want to be petted. They will meow, bunt their owners, rub against their owners' legs, and even reach out with a paw to pull their owners' hands toward them. Many cats do not like to have their tails touched; others dislike it when their feet are handled. It is very common for a cat to roll over on her back, exposing her stomach as if she wants it rubbed. Some cats will immediately attack an owner's hand with all four feet, claws extended, when he does rub her stomach. Cat-loving visitors have to be warned of this propensity. It is not clear why some cats do this. For more about cats that are aggressive when being petted, see "Aggression Toward People," below.

If an owner wants a cat to sit on his lap or next to him, he needs to remain quiet and not move around too much. Sometimes a cat will get too hot sitting or sleeping on an owner's lap and will prefer to sleep nearby instead. This is especially true of longhaired cats.

Cats that are close to their owners do respond to vocal praise and scolding, although to a lesser degree than dogs do. For instance, "No," accompanied by a loud hand clap, will certainly get most cats' attention.

Elimination Behavior

Cats appear to eliminate in daylight hours rather than at night. An owner will often notice that a cat goes to the kitty litter first thing in the morning. As with most mammals, defecation in cats is stimulated by eating. They are most likely to have a bowel movement after a meal. Cats normally have one or two bowel movements a day. Of course, the more a cat drinks, the more she will urinate. An increase of either defecation or urination can be a sign of disease.

There is a discussion of litter trays and litter in Chapter 2, page 32, and below, page 42. Owners should be aware that constipation is a fairly common problem in cats (see page 132), so it is important to be aware of a cat's normal elimination habits.

As a rule, neutered male cats and female cats squat to urinate. Unneutered males (tomcats) almost always stand with their tails raised and spray urine on an upright surface. As we said above in "Territorial Behavior," sometimes neutered males, and females neutered or not, will also spray urine. If a cat regularly sprays urine in the litter box, an owner may need to use plastic to protect the wall or any furniture that abuts a litter tray. An enclosed litter tray works well, too, but many cats will not use one.

Some Inappropriate Feline Behaviors

Aggression Toward People

An owner of an aggressive cat who had bite marks up and down his legs once coined a phrase, "the abused owner." Some cats are extremely aggressive toward people. They may attack people without seeming provocation, and have been known to knock an older person down.

There are three types of aggression displayed by cats. One kind is *predatory aggression,* which causes a cat to jump out from beneath a piece of furniture and attack a person's ankles. This usually occurs with kittens who have not

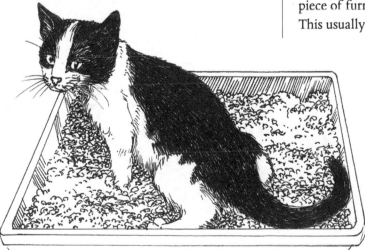

A cat squatting. This is the normal urinating posture for female cats and neutered males.

been left with their litters long enough to learn to inhibit their biting behavior. An owner can often avoid this kind of attack if he remembers to make a loud noise as he approaches the spot where the cat is hiding, or squirts the cat with water before she has an opportunity to attack. He should also be sure the cat has lots of opportunities for interactive play with a dangling object, rolling ball, windup mouse, or crinkled paper, for instance.

Redirected aggression occurs when a cat is really upset at something else. A strange cat outside the window, for example, may cause her to attack a person who just happens to be there.

The third kind of aggression is *dominant/territorial aggression,* which is similar to that in dogs. This type of aggressive cat will bite a person who pets her, but will rarely scratch a person. Dominant/aggressive cats can be treated by using the method of trying to become dominant over them. For instance, if a cat jumps on an owner's lap and then bites when the owner pats her three times, the owner should pat the cat once and then stand up, forcing her to jump down. A dominant/aggressive cat should not be allowed to rub her cheek or tail glands against her owner; the owner should just walk away.

Teaching a dominant/aggressive cat to do tricks will also increase an owner's dominance over the cat. Cats can be taught to do various tricks such as sitting, climbing a ladder, jumping through a hoop, and so forth. In general, cats can be taught better with tempting food treats (tuna fish, for example) than with praise.

As a breed, Persian cats have been found to be less aggressive than other cats.

Aggression Toward Other Cats in a Household

We spoke about the problems of territorial aggression between cats in the same household under "Territorial Behavior," above. A dominantly aggressive cat may make life miserable for another cat by preventing the use of the litter box, not allowing the other cat to eat or sleep where she wants, and so forth.

When a resident cat returns to the household after a stay at the veterinarian's, she may be treated aggressively by a formerly friendly feline housemate. This hostility may be triggered by several factors. First, cats are so smell oriented they recognize each other almost completely by scent. Therefore, a change in a cat's odor makes her seem to be a stranger to her former friend,

This cat is exhibiting dominance aggression, with ears swiveled backward, head down, rear end up, and tail curved down and fluffed slightly.

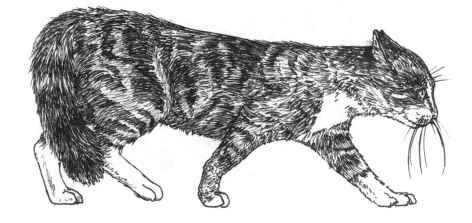

triggering an aggressive reaction. The other contributing factor may be that if the cat returning from the veterinarian's is the least bit under the weather due to anesthesia or whatever procedure she has undergone, the other cat will immediately seize the opportunity to attack.

Aggression also occurs frequently when a new cat is introduced to a household. Owners must realize that a resident cat, or cats, will probably not be pleased with a newcomer and should initially protect the new cat from aggression by isolating her. Isolate her in a room for a week; exchange litter pans daily (the new cat's and the resident cat's), and rub each cat with the same towel, especially in the cheek area. If there is no growling or other signs of aggression by either cat, it may be safe to release the new cat. Isolation is a good idea for any cat in a new house, even if she is not new to a family. This way she will be able to become used to a small space before she has the entire house, and/or the outdoors, to get used to. (Note: In Chapter 2, we speak of isolating a new cat as a means of preventing the spread of infectious or contagious disease.)

The same type of redirected aggression that may occur in a cat toward a person (see above) may occur in one cat toward another.

To reintroduce fighting cats, place both cats in carriers or cages at opposite ends of a room while the cats are fed. The cages should gradually be moved closer together until both cats are able to eat peacefully, side by side. At this point the nonaggressive cat can be allowed her freedom at mealtime, while the aggressive cat remains caged. Eventually, if both cats are able to eat in close proximity without growling or hissing, they can both be allowed their freedom. In severe cases, or if the aggression is triggered by fear, a tranquilizer may be prescribed by a veterinarian.

Destructive Behavior

Clawing of furniture and rugs is probably the most commonly seen destructive behavior in cats. Appropriate scratching posts, or devices, are helpful for many cats (see above in "Clawing Behavior"). Owners who are at home most of the time find that clapping their hands loudly and spraying a cat with water the moment she lays a paw on an inappropriate object will help, as long as she is then redirected to the scratching post. Kitty condos and other play/climbing furniture can also be used to redirect a cat's clawing instinct. Even when an owner is not home all of the time, many cats will respond to scolding and spraying and learn not to claw furniture.

We mentioned vinyl claw covers, or caps, in Chapter 2. These can be used if a cat steadfastly refuses to use a scratching post and claws the furniture instead. As we discuss in Chapter 2, if a cat is a persistent, destructive clawer, a declawing operation may be the only alternative to getting rid of her.

A second type of destructive behavior is chewing of nonfood items. Most common is wool chewing or fabric chewing, especially by Oriental breeds such as Siamese. Increasing the roughage in their diets with a high-fiber prescription diet and providing a "cat garden" of safe plants may help. Cats may eat ribbon, telephone or computer cords, plastic, or wood. If they have no tooth or gum problems and diet changes do not help, drug therapy for a compulsive problem may be necessary.

Housebreaking Problems

Elimination outside the litter box is often caused by a medical problem, so the first thing an owner should do if he is having a problem with a cat eliminating in the wrong place is to have her examined by a veterinarian.

The second major cause of house soiling in cats is lack of hygiene. Most cats simply will not use a litter box that is not clean. Owners often put a litter box in the basement, where it is out of sight and cannot be smelled, and forget to clean it regularly. Most cats prefer to urinate in one place and defecate in another, so a single cat should have two litter boxes. A cat will often refuse to use a litter box that has been soiled by another cat. If there is more than one cat in a household, the rule of thumb is to have one more litter box than the number of cats.

In multicat households, house soiling can also have a social cause. That is, one cat may frighten another whenever she approaches the litter box. A timid cat may also be frightened away by a loud noise such as a washing machine, or other distraction that occurs just as she's about to use the litter pan.

Cats will sometimes urinate directly into a bathtub or shower drain. Behaviorists speculate this may be because they always dig a hole before urinating, and a drain is a nice hole already dug for them. This behavior can also signify a medical problem; the coolness of the porcelain may feel good to a cat that is not feeling well. One way to discourage urinating in a sink or tub is to leave an inch or two of water in the tub all of the time. But remember, a cat may then find an equally unacceptable alternative!

Some cats also have location preferences and will not use a litter pan that is in the "wrong" place. An owner must turn into a detective in this case and experiment with different locations for the pan.

Covered litter pans are preferred by a small number of cats, but most cats like to be able to see in at least three directions while using a litter pan because they feel vulnerable at this time.

Preferences as to type of litter can be very strong—nine out of ten cats prefer clumping litter (fine sand that forms a clump when wet) to the plain, coarser, clay variety. Although most owners do not like this type of litter because it is messy, one of the best ways to lure a cat back to using the litter tray instead of the bathroom rug is to give her clumping litter in her pan. There are a number of mats and pads on the market today that are designed to clean a cat's paws once she has walked in clumping litter and help prevent the fine sand from being tracked all over the house.

Longhaired cats, Himalayans and Persians in particular, are apt to develop elimination problems. Behaviorists do not know why, but there has been speculation that longhairs may not like to get litter on their furry feet. Anyone who is contemplating ownership of a longhaired cat should be aware of the fact that housebreaking problems may arise.

Urine spraying can be a big problem with all cats. Unneutered male cats (tomcats) and females in heat spray continually. One out of every ten neutered males and one out of every twenty spayed females also spray from time to time. Inappropriate spraying occurs most often in multiple-cat households. There is now a product on the market made from cheek pheromones that may help deter a cat from spraying. But, because excess spraying is usually due to some kind of social stress, appropriate drugs or a redistribution of cats frequently are used to treat the problem.

Predatory Behavior

Of course, the best way to prevent a cat from hunting is to keep her indoors all of the time. Some indoor-outdoor cats are hunters and some are not. If a cat is a hunter, a breakaway collar (one which the cat can slip out of if she becomes caught on a branch or other object) with two bells, one on the top and one on the bottom, may help warn birds in some cases. One bell underneath a cat's chin often does not work because a determined cat can learn to hold the bell quiet with her chin. An owner should place bird feeders in locations where the cat can't reach them, and also make it a point not to let a hunting cat outdoors at the time the birds are most active.

How Cats Behave When They're Not Feeling Well

Even a cat that is very close to her owner will usually find a dark, small space to hide in when she is not feeling well. She often cannot be coaxed out to eat or drink. Behaviorists believe that this behavior is instinctive predator avoidance. That is, if a cat does not feel well and is unable to flee from a potential predator, she feels safer if she is well hidden. Thoughtful owners should leave the cat alone as much as possible. Of course, a pet cat cannot be allowed to remain hidden, without food or water or medical care, for more than twenty-four hours. She must be gotten out of her hiding place, forcibly, if necessary, so that an owner can assess the situation and provide veterinary care.

What to Do if a Behavior Problem Develops

If a cat develops a behavior problem the first step for an owner to take is to go to the veterinarian to be sure there is no medical reason for the cat's misbehavior. For example, a housebreaking problem could be a sign of a urinary tract disorder (see pages 54, 136–37) or hyperthyroidism (see pages 134 and 140); sudden aggressive behavior might be caused by toxoplasmosis (see pages 66–67) or a brain tumor.

Once a medical cause for the misbehavior has been ruled out, a veterinarian may be able to prescribe medication intended to modify the behavior. Or he might suggest behavior therapy and put the owner in touch with a board-certified veterinary behaviorist, or someone certified by The Animal Behavior Society, who has passed requirements to practice animal behavior modification. There are very few cat trainers available to owners for advice.

Owner Responsibilities

Cat ownership is a great deal less onerous than dog ownership. But although cats are able to spend considerable time alone at home, a potential cat owner must be sure that he provides the proper environment for a cat to thrive in.

A cat that is left alone for hours at a time should have an appropriate clawing device and also some type of play furniture and toys for exercise. She needs clean litter and fresh drinking water. If she is allowed to snack on dry food during the day, her food bowl should contain plenty of food.

Besides providing for her physical needs, a cat owner needs to give his pet loving attention and playtime when he arrives home in the evening. As we pointed out earlier, because cats are crepuscular by nature, the evening hours are particularly appropriate for playtime.

Part Two

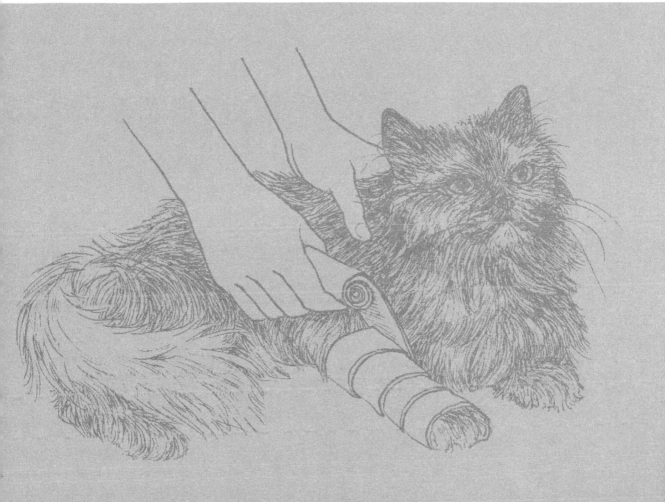

A Sick
or Injured Cat

Accidents

and Medical

Emergencies

Most emergency situations involving cats are usually due either to accidental injury or to illness. Emergencies due to accidental injury may include *trauma,* such as a bad fall, hard blow, or being hit by a moving vehicle. In these cases a cat may suffer from fractures, concussion, or other internal injuries. *Lacerations and wounds* can be emergency situations if there is a lot of blood loss, and bite wounds from other cats can cause abscesses and serious infections such as pyothorax (see page 53). It is an emergency situation if a cat eats a *poisoned rat or mouse* or ingests a harmful household substance such as antifreeze, human medication, or some poisonous plants. Because of their propensity to play with string or thread, both kittens and cats often *swallow* this type of material and these "linear" foreign bodies can obstruct and/or cut through a cat's intestines. A cat can be accidentally *burned, electrocuted,* or suffer from *smoke inhalation;* in rare cases, cats can also *drown.* An *illness* may be an emergency if it is sudden and acute, or an ongoing illness can become an emergency for many reasons.

Avoiding Accidents

An important thing for a cat owner to bear in mind is that no matter how smart a kitten or cat may be, he has no concept of potential danger, especially if he has lived in a protected environment all of his life. It is up to an owner to think for her pet and try to make sure he is protected from dangerous situations as far as is possible.

When an owner is aware of the types of accidental emergency situations a kitten or cat can get himself into, she can use her common sense to take steps to avoid them. By anticipating danger for a kitten or cat, just as she would for a human toddler, an owner can prevent many emergency situations from arising.

"Kitten-Proofing"

One of the best things an owner of a new kitten (or even an adult cat that is new to the household) can do to protect a pet from accidental injury in the home is to take time to carefully examine the space the kitten will be living in, from the animal's point of view, and remove any potential hazards.

For the first few days, many owners find it is best to confine a new kitten or cat to one room so he can become used to the household and its other residents gradually. A frightened new kitten may prefer a safe dark space at first, so any room where he can find a nice big piece of furniture to get underneath may suit him best. Food and water dishes and a litter pan should be placed nearby. As soon as the kitten begins to emerge from his hiding place and make friends

with the humans in the household, it is usually safe to allow him the run of the house.

In general, kittens do not seem to suffer from much discomfort from teething, but they may still chew on things, especially dangling cords or wires. If a kitten chews on a plugged-in electric wire, he can easily be electrocuted, so it is safest to unplug electric wires when no one is around to watch a kitten, at least until an owner is sure the kitten will not chew on them.

As we mentioned above, almost all kittens and cats are intrigued by anything long and thin such as string, thread, or yarn (tinsel is especially tempting at Christmastime, and can be lethal). A thorough search should be made of the house before a kitten or cat is allowed complete freedom, to be sure all such objects are securely put away in a drawer or behind a closed door. Remember, it is not enough to put them up on a high surface or cubbyhole—cats can jump high and are able to squeeze into small spaces.

Trauma

Because cats cannot be confined with a fence to a yard or run, the only way to avoid the possible trauma from their being hit by a car, motorcycle, or bicycle is to keep them indoors or teach them to walk with a harness and leash. As we mentioned in Chapter 2, indoor-only cats not only lead full and happy lives, but almost always live longer than their roaming cousins.

When riding in a car, a cat should always be in a sturdy carrying case so he cannot jump out of a suddenly opened door or window (see Chapter 2, page 17, for a discussion of types of carrying cases). When secured with a seat belt, a carrying case may help prevent serious injury in case of a car accident.

Outdoor cats are often injured by cars in a

different fashion. On a cold night a cat will sometimes get underneath a car hood to sleep on top of the warm engine. When the engine is started in the morning, the cat can be severely injured by the fan and engine belts.

Kittens and cats are especially prone to traumatic injury due to falls from windows. Known as the "high-rise syndrome," this can occur in the country or suburbs as well as a city apartment. A fall from a second-story window onto a flagstone path or tiled terrace can be just as damaging as one from a fourth-floor apartment window. Cats and kittens are particularly apt to become fascinated with an insect or bird flying by and forget where they are. Neither kittens nor grown cats should ever be left alone in an upstairs room with open, unscreened windows. Window bars do little to deter a cat, by the way, as most cats can squeeze right through them.

A study of the records of "high-rise" cats admitted to the Bobst Hospital of The Animal Medical Center in New York City revealed some very interesting facts about falling cats. The most serious injuries and the highest mortality rates occurred in cats who fell between five and nine floors. Cats who fell four floors or less and cats who fell ten or more floors had less serious injuries. Cats falling from lower floors are not falling as fast as cats falling from greater than five floors. After five floors, it is predictable that a falling cat has reached terminal velocity—that is, there will be no further increase in speed no matter how great the distance. It appears that cats falling from ten floors or greater have time to right themselves and fall in a position similar to parachutists in free fall, with the legs spread out to the side and the body parallel to the ground. When a cat hits the ground in this position, much of the shock is absorbed by his flexible rib cage and abdomen. The most serious injury in "high-rise" cats is pneumothorax (collapsed lungs with free air in the chest cavity). This is an emergency; the air must be removed by a veterinarian to allow the lungs to re-expand. But it is very possible to save a cat who has fallen great distances. Two cats who survived in New York City fell thirty-two and forty-six floors.

Kittens' curiosity can also get them into trouble if they dart, unseen, into open closets, bureau drawers, and other spaces where they can become trapped. Refrigerators and clothes dryers are also hazardous; young kittens, especially, often climb into them and can suffocate or be killed if they are not discovered. Some adult cats never outgrow the tendency to get into small spaces; not only should owners be aware of this, but any

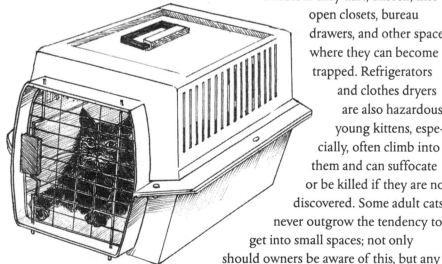

Cat in a carrying case. The best and safest type of cat carrier is made of rigid, waterproof material with wire on one side and plenty of air vents.

caretakers should be told always to check to see where a cat is before turning on the dryer or leaving the house.

Poisoning

Cats are not as subject to accidental poisoning as dogs because they are apt to be more choosy about what they eat. But there are exceptions. Kittens' curiosity may lead them to sample something an adult cat would not, so owners should be especially careful to keep any harmful substances out of their reach. Again, it is important to remember cats' ability to reach things, so any potentially poisonous substances should not only be put away, but must be securely closed.

Many common household chemicals are poisonous to cats as well as humans, but most do not appeal to cats because of their foul smell or taste. An exception to this is *antifreeze,* which has a sweetish taste that is irresistible to cats. Antifreeze contains ethylene glycol, a highly toxic chemical fatal to cats. Antifreeze should be kept in tightly closed containers, and extreme care needs to be taken that no radiator fluid containing antifreeze has leaked onto a driveway or garage floor. This is especially important for an indoor-outdoor cat, but even an indoor-only cat may venture into an attached garage. A cat that is suspected of ingesting antifreeze needs *immediate* veterinary care to prevent kidney failure and eventual death. A safer antifreeze made with propylene glycol is now available commercially. Pet owners may want to consider using it as an alternative.

Rat poison is another insidious danger for cats. Although they are not apt to eat the poison itself, they can be poisoned if they catch and bite or eat a poisoned mouse or rat. Rat poisons contain a substance called warfarin, or similar chemicals, that interferes with a cat's blood-clotting ability and blocks the production of vitamin K. A cat that has ingested rat poison may become anemic, have trouble breathing, suffer from nosebleeds, internal bleeding, and bruising. Prompt treatment with vitamin K injections and blood transfusions will usually help.

Cats are particularly sensitive to medications and can suffer from *drug intoxication* if they eat or drink human medications, especially those containing acetaminophen. A cat who has ingested acetaminophen doses as small as a simple pill may develop methemoglobinemia, a condition in which blood hemoglobin is changed so that it doesn't carry oxygen. Poisoned cats will exhibit difficult breathing, dark blue tongue and mucous membranes, and a swollen face. Immediate treatment is necessary to prevent fatality. *No medication is safe to give to a cat without veterinary supervision.*

Cats often play with, and chew, houseplants and will play with fallen berries and leaves. However, *plant poisoning* is usually not a serious problem because the bitter or foul taste of most plants prevents a cat from ingesting a great deal. The greatest problem can be a potentially dangerous swelling of the mucous membranes of a cat's mouth and throat. Dieffenbachia, or dumbcane, contains a particularly large amount of a substance that can cause swelling of the mucous membranes, and mistletoe and holly berries can make a cat quite sick if he eats enough of them. Japanese yew can be fatal to cats and members of the lily family can cause kidney failure.

If a kitten or cat is known to have eaten anything potentially poisonous, an owner should immediately call a veterinarian. If a veterinarian cannot be reached, call the ASPCA National Animal Poison Control Center at 1-800-548-2423.

4

This center is manned by veterinarians and board-certified toxicologists and is open twenty-four hours a day, every day. A $30 consultation fee is payable by credit card. If possible, an owner should have information available about the substance ingested. Immediate action can often prevent permanent health damage and even death.

For free nonemergency information about pesticides concerning both animals and people, call The National Pesticide Telecommunications Network (NPTN) at 1-800-858-7378. At this number, graduate scientists will answer inquiries about lawn-care and gardening products, pest-control products, and so forth, as they might affect both pets and people. This service, available from 6:30 A.M. to 4:30 P.M., Pacific time, seven days a week, excluding holidays, is a cooperative effort of Oregon State University and the U.S. Environmental Protection Agency. See also "Drug Poisoning/Intoxication," page 57, and Appendix A, page 145.

Heat Prostration

The most frequent reason a cat suffers from heat prostration is because he is left in a carrying case in a parked car during warm weather. On a sunny day when the temperature is in the seventies, it takes only a few minutes of sunshine on the car for the interior to heat up to over a hundred degrees, even if the windows are partially open. The poor ventilation in a carrying case combined with the heat in the car leads to heat prostration, which develops very quickly in cats because of their small size and inefficient means of cooling their bodies. The only way cats have to cool themselves down is by panting to allow moisture to evaporate from their mouths.

A cat may also suffer from heat prostration

if he is closed in a small, hot, poorly ventilated room. Brachycephalic cats are especially prone to heat prostration because of the malformation of their faces and noses.

If a cat does appear to have difficulty breathing, or collapses from the heat, he must be rushed to a veterinarian immediately in order to save his life. More about heat prostration on pages 57–58.

Some Feline Medical Emergencies

As we said above, an ongoing illness can develop into an emergency for various reasons. A severe medical problem that occurs suddenly is also an emergency situation. Following are some commonly occurring feline medical emergencies. In most instances there are no effective home first aid steps that can or should be taken, and prompt veterinary care is necessary.

Bleeding

BLOODY DIARRHEA OR STOOL

When a cat is passing normal stools or diarrhea containing streaks or flecks of blood, it is not a severe emergency. If, however, a cat passes a lot of blood rectally, veterinary attention should be sought immediately. There is no first aid for serious blood loss in the stool.

BLOOD IN THE URINE

Bloody urine is usually a sign of a urinary tract infection such as *bacterial cystitis,* and is not a serious emergency. If the urine is very dark or blood clots are passed, it is a sign of profuse bleeding, which requires immediate veterinary attention. There is no first aid for serious blood loss in the urine.

VOMITING BLOOD

If fluid is being vomited, vomiting is infrequent, or there are only flecks or streaks of blood in the vomitus, it is not a serious emergency. If, however, there is a profuse amount of blood thrown up or if there are blood clots present, it can indicate serious bleeding in a cat's stomach. There is no first aid for this condition and immediate veterinary help is necessary. Oral medication should *not* be given if a cat is vomiting blood.

SPONTANEOUS BRUISING, NOSE BLEEDS

Bruising can be difficult for an owner to recognize because of a cat's haircoat. If there are purple splotches on a cat's stomach it can be a sign of a clotting disorder. Bleeding from the nose can also be very serious and can occur from a clotting disorder, possibly from rat poison. Small purple or red spots on the insides of a cat's ears or on his gums may indicate a low platelet count, or some other type of bleeding disorder. A cat can bleed into internal cavities, such as the chest, or abdomen, which can cause severe problems. Bruising of any sort should be considered serious and veterinary care sought.

Breathing Problems

If a cat has difficulty breathing he may be suffering from *feline bronchial asthma,* a condition very similar to human asthma. This can be the result of an allergic reaction to some airborne pollen, dust from the environment or cat litter, and so forth. It can be a serious or life-threatening emergency and veterinary care should begin immediately. Asthma in cats can be controlled but never cured completely. Cats with asthma usually have a history of coughing, so

owners should pay attention to this rather uncommon symptom in cats.

Whenever a cat is having difficulty breathing it should be considered a severe emergency. Breathing difficulty can be caused by *cardiomyopathy* (see below), *feline infectious peritonitis* (*FIP*—see page 60), *pneumonia* (see below), or a serious chest injury that produces *pneumothorax*. If a cat has had a serious chest injury such as a fall, being hit by a car, or an invasive chest wound, he will have great difficulty breathing and may have bluish mucous membranes (cyanosis) as well. This is a severe emergency that requires immediate veterinary help. Cyanosis is a sign of insufficient oxygen.

Cardiovascular Emergencies

Cardiomyopathy

Cats do not suffer from cholesterol problems or heart attacks as people do. The most commonly seen feline heart disease is disease of the heart muscle and can take several forms. A cat can have cardiomyopathy for years before symptoms surface. *Hypertrophic cardiomyopathy* (*HCM*) causes the heart to fail suddenly. A cat will develop fluid in his lungs (pulmonary edema) and will have difficulty breathing. *Dilated (congestive) cardiomyopathy* often creates a buildup of fluid in a cat's chest cavity outside his lungs, causing the lungs to collapse. Cats with heart failure will be very quiet, reluctant to move, and may exhibit difficulty breathing. These cats require immediate veterinary help.

Collapse

Collapse, or unconsciousness, can be due to a number of conditions that are described in this chapter such as: shock following a traumatic injury; an ongoing systemic or metabolic disease; severe blood loss; difficulty breathing; poisoning; anemia; or seizures. In some cases, a cat may even lose consciousness. In all cases, a cat that has collapsed or become unconscious must be evaluated by a veterinarian right away.

Diarrhea

Cats do not suffer from diarrhea as frequently as dogs do. If a cat has an occasional bout of diarrhea it is usually not serious and may be the result of injudicious eating of prey, for instance. Exceptions are bloody diarrhea (see above), if it lasts for longer than twenty-four hours, and/or if the diarrhea is accompanied by vomiting or other symptoms of illness such as fever, loss of appetite, and signs of pain or illness. Then it may be a sign of poisoning (see page 50), or a systemic illness or infection.

Hypoglycemia

Hypoglycemia, or low blood sugar, usually occurs in cats that are undergoing insulin treatment for *diabetes mellitus* (see Glossary), and is characterized by several different signs. A cat with this condition may be weak and confused. He may not respond to his name, and pace and wander aimlessly. If hypoglycemia is allowed to go on for too long, *seizures* and eventually *coma* will follow.

A cat with hypoglycemia may have an acute onset of seizures or convulsions. During a seizure a cat will roll over on his side, make rapid jaw movements, salivate profusely, let go of bowel and bladder, and shake his limbs violently.

With hypoglycemia, first aid treatment may help. Honey, syrup, or sugar water may reverse the problem for a cat that begins to become confused or weak, but only if it is given at the first sign of a problem, before seizures or collapse occur. Approximately one tablespoon of something containing sugar should be spooned or dropped into a cat's mouth, a little at a time. Do not try to give anything orally if the cat is unconscious! Even with proper treatment there may sometimes be brain damage. A veterinary checkup should be given once the cat is stabilized. Kittens who are not eating may also become hypoglycemic. Never allow a small kitten to be fasted for a prolonged period.

Pneumonia

Unlike with other animals, pneumonia can occur in cats without any preceding symptoms such as coughing. The first signs of pneumonia in a cat can be severe, life-threatening, labored breathing, collapse, and bluish mucous membranes (cyanosis). This is an emergency condition requiring immediate veterinary help.

Pyometra

Pyometra is a surgical emergency that occurs in older, unspayed, female cats. It is an infection of the uterus and has variable signs and symptoms. Some cats may show only a gradually enlarging abdomen, while others may also show signs of systemic illness, including anorexia, fever, depression, vomiting, or diarrhea. Surgical removal of the uterus is the only treatment.

Pyothorax

This is a condition arising from a raging infection in a cat's chest cavity. A cat with pyothorax is extremely sick and probably is running a fever. Because of fluid in the chest cavity, he will have severe difficulty breathing (dyspnea) and will be very depressed.

The infection is caused by either a penetrating wound or a systemic spreading of bacteria in a cat's bloodstream due to a simple bite or puncture wound. This is a life-threatening condition and requires immediate veterinary intervention.

Seizures/Convulsions

Seizures are not as common in cats as they are in dogs, but they can occur and are usually brought about by a medical condition such as hypoglycemia (see above), or an inflammatory disease of the brain. Idiopathic (no known cause) epilepsy is also possible.

If a seizure is short and the cat then returns to normal it is not a serious emergency. However, if a cat has several continuous seizures that last a long time (status epilecticus), or is having multiple seizures (sequence clustering) he may die or have permanent brain damage due to hypoxia (loss of oxygen to the tissues). Hospitalization and intravenous administration of various anticonvulsants are necessary—this is an extremely serious condition. An owner's detailed history of the onset of seizures is invaluable to a veterinarian in making a diagnosis and decision about how to treat the underlying cause of a seizure.

Urinary Emergencies

A cat that is straining to urinate may be suffering from *feline lower urinary tract disease* (FLUTD, formerly known as FUS). Other signs of this disease may be frequent licking of the genital region, bloody urine, and urinating outside the litter pan. Some cats show no initial symptoms of FLUTD and simply become very ill. If the urethra becomes obstructed the cat will be in obvious pain, may vomit and lose his appetite, and will show signs of straining to urinate. Male cats are affected more often than females. If it is not treated promptly, the condition may lead to a dangerous level of potassium elevation in a cat's body, which can cause heart problems and death.

The cause of FLUTD in cats is still being debated. It does not appear to be caused by an infection and may be related to a dietary mineral imbalance, urine too high in pH (alkaline urine), and/or some inherent predisposing factor. There are prescription diets on the market that can help prevent recurrences of this problem. Sometimes a surgical procedure called a perineal urethrostomy to shorten, straighten, and widen a male cat's urethra is necessary to stop the problem.

Vomiting

All cats vomit occasionally and some vomit two or three times a week without signs of illness.

If a cat vomits but seems to feel well otherwise it is usually not an emergency. If the vomiting is preceded by retching and the resulting vomitus is tubelike and contains hair, it is a hair ball and can be safely ignored (for steps to help prevent hair balls, see page 140). If, however, there is a lot of blood in the vomitus (see "Vomiting Blood," above), if it persists for more than twenty-four hours or is accompanied by diarrhea, fever, abdominal distension, obvious discomfort or pain, weakness, loss of appetite, or listlessness, it may be a symptom of a number of different conditions. Veterinary help should be sought right away in any of these cases. If a cat vomits

Shock

Cats can be in shock from trauma (from a fall, car injury, etc.), severe bleeding or hemorrhaging, heart disease, or systemic illness. Shock is a collapse of the cardiovascular system and is characterized by: rapid heartbeat; confusion; collapse; weak pulse; and pale mucous membranes. Normally, a cat's gums and the insides of her cheeks are bright pink. However, the mucous membranes can vary in normal color. An owner should check a cat's mucous membranes when the animal is well, in order to see how they look. To do this, lift up a corner of a cat's lip and examine the gums and mucous membranes of the mouth. If they are pale pink, the cat may be stressed, in mild shock, or may be anemic; if they are white, the problem is serious. If shock has been brought about by severe blood loss it is called *hemorrhagic shock*. Heavy fluid loss can lead to *hypovolemic shock*.

A cat suspected of being in shock should be kept quiet and warm and have immediate veterinary care. If shock is not treated promptly a cat will die.

frequently and is losing weight, the problem should also be investigated.

Accidental Feline Emergencies

In general, the best treatment an owner can provide for a cat suffering from an accidental injury is to get him to a veterinarian right away. It is foolish and dangerous to waste precious time trying to give emergency first aid, and often whatever measures are taken won't help and may harm a cat. If there are appropriate first aid steps, they are included here.

External Bleeding

Because a cat's blood volume makes up only about 6 percent of his total body weight, blood loss is of particular concern in cats. Bleeding or hemorrhaging from any part of a cat's body is an emergency whether it is acute, profuse bleeding, or chronic, continuous blood loss. The best way to determine if the bleeding is serious is to check for signs of shock (see above) or anemia.

Bleeding from the Nose or Mouth

This can be life-threatening if bleeding is profuse. Cold compresses or ice packs can slow the bleeding but are very difficult to apply. Emergency veterinary treatment should be sought immediately.

Bleeding from the Skin

Cuts or wounds on a cat's skin surface will cause some bleeding although it is usually not severe. If a wound is deep it can puncture a vein or blood vessel beneath the skin surface and bleeding will be more profuse. This is most likely to happen in cats if the wound is in the neck or leg area (see below). Apply pressure by hand to slow the bleeding using a clean cloth or bandage (see illustration, below). If the area can be bandaged, a compression bandage should be used (see illustration, below).

Foot and Leg Bleeding

Cats walk lightly and do not often cut their feet. But if they do, lacerations of the footpads bleed a great deal. Cats' footpads consist of spongy tissue and even after bleeding has stopped, cuts often bleed again as soon as a cat steps on his foot. To prevent continuous blood loss from a footpad laceration, a pressure bandage should be used.

More serious, spurting arterial bleeding can occur if a cat cuts the small artery that runs up the leg right behind the footpads. This is not a common injury in cats, but it can occur if a cat is caught and bitten by a dog, for instance, or is hit by a moving vehicle. This type of bleeding should be stopped with a pressure bandage placed around the entire foot and lower leg. *The use of tourniquets is not advised.* They can easily cause the loss of a limb due to inadequate blood supply and do not stop bleeding as well as pressure.

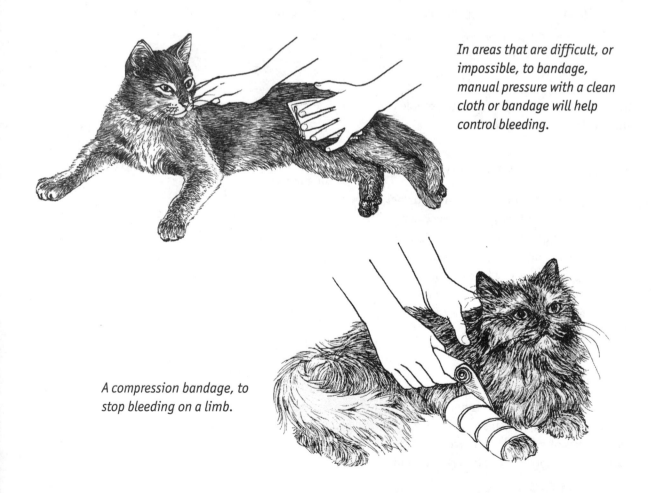

In areas that are difficult, or impossible, to bandage, manual pressure with a clean cloth or bandage will help control bleeding.

A compression bandage, to stop bleeding on a limb.

Broken Bones

A cat can break any one of the hundreds of bones in his body. A cat with a suspected fracture should be kept quiet, treated for shock (see above), and moved as little as possible. Pick the cat up by his chest or stomach and place him in a carrying case, carton, or even a clean litter tray, and take him to the veterinarian (see page 17). Splints or other means of immobilizing an injured limb usually cause more discomfort and pain to a cat than leaving it alone.

Burns

Cats are rarely burned with fire, but they can fall into a tub of scalding water. More often, they can be burned when scalding water or hot grease falls on them. This can cause diffuse burns that can be extremely serious. No first aid is recommended, but prompt medical treatment is necessary.

Drug Poisoning/Intoxication

Cats should never be given any medication without a veterinarian's advice. Even drugs that are generally considered safe for other species, such as aspirin, acetaminophen, tranquilizers, and so forth can cause serious problems in cats. Cats are not apt to swallow anything unfamiliar, but if a cat should swallow any human medications or drugs such as marijuana, hashish, or hallucinogenics, it is an emergency. If an owner is sure a cat has ingested medicine or other drugs that are not caustic, she should get the material out of the cat quickly by inducing vomiting. Hydrogen peroxide given orally with a spoon will cause a cat to vomit and will not harm him. The cat should be

seen by a veterinarian right away to be sure no drug remains in his body and to check for any side effects. See also Appendix A, page 145.

Electrocution

Kittens, which may chew electric wires, are much more apt to suffer from electrocution than adult cats. Electrocution may be mild and there may be very few signs, but it usually results in shock and significant pulmonary edema (fluid in the lungs), causing labored, difficult breathing (dyspnea). Cyanosis (blue mucous membranes) may be present, as may shock (see above). A kitten must be treated right away with diuretics and oxygen to save his life. If an owner comes home and finds a kitten lying on his side unable to move and having difficulty breathing, she should suspect electrocution. This is true even if visible burns are not obvious in the mouth or on the tongue.

Eye Injuries

Cats' eyes are often injured in fights with other cats. Any eye injury must be treated quickly and appropriately to prevent permanent damage. No first aid, such as putting water on the eye, should be attempted as it will upset the delicate eye membranes and will do more harm than good.

Heat Prostration

We spoke about heat prostration earlier in this chapter. Any cat that regularly has difficulty breathing such as an extremely brachycephalic cat, one that is severely overweight, or a cat with a heart problem will be at greater risk from heat prostration if he becomes overheated or overexerts.

If a cat is suffering from heat prostration he will breathe noisily with his tongue hanging out and may have thick foam and saliva in his mouth. His body temperature will be very high and he may be in shock (see "Shock," page 55). It is imperative to quickly cool a cat that is suffering from heat prostration. It is all right to try to cool a cat by misting him all over with a spray bottle, but it is best to rush him to the veterinarian as quickly as possible so that he can be cooled and receive medication to prevent brain damage from the heat and hypoxia (deficiency of oxygen). If the cat has blue mucous membranes, there may be an airway obstruction from thick saliva in the back of his throat. If an owner can safely open the cat's mouth and clear the saliva with a paper towel or gauze square, it may save the cat's life. The leading cause of death from heat prostration is cardiovascular collapse, shock, and a condition known as DIC, a bleeding disorder caused by prolonged excess body heat. DIC often starts with bleeding from the nose and progresses to profuse hemorrhaging. Once it has begun, there is usually nothing that can be done to save the cat.

Contagious

and

Infectious

Feline

Diseases

Although cats are susceptible to a number of infectious and contagious diseases just as all other mammals are, for many years research into feline diseases and the development of preventive medicines for cats took a backseat to the study of canine diseases. Now, however, with the burgeoning growth of cat ownership, knowledge of cat diseases and how to prevent and treat them has grown by leaps and bounds.

Infectious diseases are caused when a cat's body is invaded by a disease-producing entity or entities such as bacteria, fungi, protozoans, parasites, or viruses. Contagious diseases are infectious diseases that can be passed from one cat to another. Thus, contagious diseases are always infectious, but not all infectious diseases are contagious (that is, able to be "caught" by a cat from another cat). In general, bacterial diseases are less contagious than viral diseases, which are usually very contagious.

Contagious diseases can be transmitted

from one cat to another by various means. These include direct contact with an infected cat or with her urine, feces, saliva, or blood; or the inhaling of airborne viruses or bacteria, which does not require direct contact between cats. Some infectious diseases are transmitted by an intermediate host such as a parasite. Viruses and bacteria can also be carried on people's hands and clothing, shoes in particular.

Fortunately, routine immunizations are almost entirely able to prevent the majority of feline infectious viral diseases. Most parasites can also be avoided by the use of preventive medications. Diseases that cannot be prevented can usually be successfully treated, providing the treatment is begun as soon as symptoms appear.

Infectious Viral Diseases Against Which Cats Can Be Immunized

Feline Infectious Peritonitis (FIP)

FIP is caused by a feline coronavirus and is a very strange disease. Like FeLV and FIV, the FIP virus is not highly contagious among cats but very young neonatal kittens may be highly susceptible to it. It is generally believed that most cats with FIP are infected early in life and the virus may be dormant in these cats for a very long time (months to many years). What eventually activates the virus is not understood at the present time. Because of the susceptibility of very young kittens, this virus is a significant problem in catteries with infected queens.

Coronavirus does not appear to directly attack a cat's organs. Rather, a combination of the vitrus and antibodies to the virus produced by the cat himself form complexes that circulate through the cat's bloodstream and eventually lodge in the blood vessels and tissues. These immune complexes then stimulate an inflammatory reaction that damages or destroys the tissues in which the immune complexes came to rest. In a very real sense, the cat's immune system is responsible for most of the disease. There are also milder strains of coronavirus (enteric coronavirus) that cause only minor intestinal disease. It is unclear whether these are less virulent forms of the same coronavirus or a different coronavirus.

Like FeLV, FIP can produce a variety of syndromes in cats. The type of disease varies with the age of the cat, virulence of the virus, the organs in which immune complexes lodge, and possibly, susceptibility of the cat. A common syndrome seen in kittens and young adults is called "wet," or effusive FIP. In this syndrome, the lining of the chest and/or abdominal cavities becomes inflamed. A high-protein, viscous watery fluid builds up in the chest or abdomen, causing difficult breathing or abdominal swelling. Accompanying signs include fever, vomiting, diarrhea, anorexia, and rapid loss of condition. This syndrome is usually quickly fatal.

In middle-aged or older cats, FIP is most often seen in the "dry," or granulomatous form. In this form, chronic, granulomatous inflammation destroys the affected organ. These cats can virtually have any symptoms, including jaundice, kidney swelling and failure, brain swelling and seizures, vomiting, diarrhea, anorexia, weight loss, and fever. In other cats, FIP may produce a "fading kitten" syndrome, lameness from joint inflammation, or chronic respiratory problems.

Testing for FIP is problematic because we only have a blood test for coronavirus antibodies. An antibody test cannot accurately separate an exposed or immune animal from a currently infected animal. Theories about high antibody titers being more indicative of infection than lower antibody titers do not apply very well in individual cases and the test is often misinterpreted. The presence of enteric coronavirus, which cross-reacts with FIP virus, adds further confusion to the situation. It is the opinion of the authors that cats should not be euthanized *only* because of a high coronavirus antibody titer. The titer can be helpful when interpreted along with other blood tests, fluid analysis, cytology, or classic signs and symptoms.

FIP usually carries a poor prognosis because there are no specific therapies for this disease. Anti-inflammatory drugs can provide some relief in cats with "dry" FIP, and other symptomatic treatments may help for a while. The "wet" form of FIP is very resistant to therapeutic intervention.

A new FIP vaccine has recently been developed, but this vaccine is somewhat controversial. The vaccine is administered intranasally to stimulate immunity at the portal of entry of the virus. Because the FIP disease is produced in part by the body's systemic immune response, this is probably a better vaccination attempt than giving an injection to stimulate systemic immunity. The vaccine should not be given until sixteen weeks of age. This is part of the controversy with this vaccine. Since many, or most, cats are infected as newborns, this may be too late to protect them. The complicated technology of this vaccine does not, however, allow earlier administration.

Feline Immunodeficiency Virus (FIV—formerly called feline T-lymphotropic lentivirus, FTLV)

FIV is a cat retrovirus that is contagious to cats, but not to dogs and humans. Like FeLV, this virus is not highly contagious among cats but can be transmitted among those with intimate social contacts. The primary mode of transmission is through bite wounds and is, therefore, most commonly seen in male cats and cats who fight with other cats. There may be other modes of transmission, however.

Like other retroviruses, FIV has a lengthy incubation period from infection to onset of symptoms. FIV is generally less aggressive than FeLV, but still will kill most cats eventually. Cancers and tumors are not caused by FIV, but serious immune-deficiency and bone marrow suppression occurs in infected cats.

There is no vaccine and no specific treatment available for FIV. Just as with FeLV, a very sensitive test is available and this can be used to limit the spread of the disease. New cats should not be introduced into households with uninfected cats until the new cat is found to be free of FIV. Outdoor cats and indoor-outdoor cats should be tested periodically and, if positive, should be isolated from uninfected cats or removed from the household.

Feline Leukemia Virus (FeLV)

The feline leukemia virus is one of the most devastating of all feline infectious diseases. The virus is classified as a retrovirus, the same type of virus as the feline immunodeficiency virus (FIV) and the human immunodeficiency virus (HIV). It is important to emphasize that these viruses are species-specific—FeLV and FIV cannot infect humans or dogs and HIV cannot infect cats or dogs. FeLV is a contagious virus between cats but is not as highly contagious as the upper respiratory viruses (see below). Casual contact between cats will not usually transmit the virus, but living together in the same house increases the risk of disease transmission over time. For this reason, uninfected cats should not be housed with infected cats.

As with other retroviruses, there may be a considerable time period (many years) from infection to development of disease symptoms. The FeLV virus can produce a variety of disease syndromes in cats. This is unpredictable from cat to cat. Cats infected with FeLV may develop cancers called lymphoma, lymphosarcoma, or leukemia, depending on the organs affected. Leukemia means cancerous lymphocytes circulating in the bloodstream. Lymphoma/lymphosarcoma are solid tumors affecting a cat's lymph nodes, spleen, intestines, anterior chest cavity, kidneys, liver, brain, and/or virtually any other body organ. Chemotherapy and/or radiation may help some cats with FeLV-induced cancer, but the eventual prognosis is not good.

The FeLV virus can also produce a syndrome of immune deficiency, in which a cat becomes unable to protect himself from other infectious agents, bacteria, protozoans, fungi, or viruses. In these infected cats, death usually occurs from secondary infections. Antibiotics and other medications may help for a while, but none of the anti-infective drugs work very well without the body's normal immune system.

The third syndrome seen in FeLV-infected cats is severe bone marrow suppression. In these cats, the bone marrow, which is responsible for manufacturing red blood cells (to carry oxygen), neutrophils (white blood cells that help fight infection), and platelets (small cells that help blood to clot), is suppressed and natural cell production is interrupted. A syndrome called *pancytopenia* (decrease in all blood cells) is seen, leaving the patient anemic, unable to fight infection, and unable to clot blood normally. There is no effec-

tive treatment for this syndrome and death eventually intervenes.

Because of the serious nature of this disease and poor available treatment, an owner must focus on prevention. There are very sensitive tests available that can detect the FeLV virus in cats long before they show disease symptoms. A new cat should not be introduced into a household with uninfected cats until the newcomer has been tested for FeLV. Outdoor cats and indoor-outdoor cats should be periodically tested according to a veterinarian's advice. FeLV positive cats should be isolated from uninfected cats or removed from the household. This virus is not very persistent in the environment and common household disinfectants, including dilute bleach solution, will kill the virus in the environment.

There are several FeLV vaccines available but there is still a lot of controversy about their use. There are side effects from the use of these vaccines in many cats. The benefit of FeLV protection versus the risk of these side effects is situational, depending mostly on a particular cat's lifestyle. This issue should be discussed with a veterinarian before a decision about vaccination is made. Most veterinarians will not recommend the vaccination for cats who are exclusively indoor cats. For these cats, the best protection is care when introducing new cats into the household. The issue is more complex for outdoor and indoor-outdoor cats. One rare side effect of the FeLV vaccine that has recently come to light is creation of a cancer called fibrosarcoma at the injection site. This is a very aggressive tumor that is probably not caused by the killed FeLV virus in the vaccine. Rather, it is probably caused by a chemical, called an adjuvant, which is added to the vaccine to stimulate the proper immune response to the FeLV virus. This side effect is rare, occurring in one in 5,000–10,000 cats, but can be fatal. Other vaccine side effects include immune system dysfunction, bone marrow suppression, and systemic illness.

Rabies

This ancient, fatal viral disease occurs throughout the world. While it can affect any warm-blooded mammal, most rabies in the United States is carried by bats, skunks, foxes, and raccoons. Chance encounters with these animals are the most common source of rabies in dogs and cats. While dogs were once the subject of most rabies legislation, rabid cats, while rare, outnumber rabid dogs and many municipalities now require rabies vaccination for cats.

There is no cure for rabies and the disease is always fatal. Concern about rabies is focused mostly on the public health aspect of the disease. The virus is transmitted primarily by animal bites with the virus present in the biting animal's saliva. The incubation period of the rabies virus varies tremendously and can range anywhere from one week up to a year. However, the presence of the virus in the infected animal's saliva occurs late in the infection, within ten days of death from the disease. This is why biting animals must be confined or observed for ten days after biting a person. If the animal is still healthy and alive ten days later, then the rabies virus was presumably not in the saliva at the time of the bite.

The most common sign of rabies in cats is neurologic impairment of a limb where a wild animal bite occurred. The virus travels up the nerves to the brain and eventually reaches the salivary glands. Therefore, any neurologic manifestation is possible, including behavioral changes, seizures, cognitive disorders, and difficulty swallowing.

Vaccination is the best method of rabies prevention. Kittens should be vaccinated at three to four months of age (depending on local laws). The first vaccine is good for one year. After that, boosters are usually good for three years. Because killed rabies virus vaccines contain an adjuvant just as the FeLV vaccine does, the same problem of vaccination-induced sarcoma can occur in cats (see FeLV, above). It is more difficult to avoid this with rabies vaccine because of laws requiring the vaccination. A nonadjuvant vaccine for cats is being developed at this time.

Upper Respiratory Infections (URI's)

The two feline upper respiratory infections that have the most severe symptoms are *calicivirus* and *rhinotracheitis*. These viruses are included in routine immunizations. Two milder upper respiratory infections, *pneumonitis* and *reovirus* are not usually part of a kitten's or cat's regular immunization series. Pneumonitis is caused by chlamydia, a bacterialike organism. All four URI's are highly contagious. Sometimes cats that have recovered from calicivirus or rhinotracheitis become carriers of the diseases and can infect other cats.

Signs of all four URI's include sneezing, runny eyes and nose. Cats with reovirus will normally present no other symptoms, will not have a fever, and will continue to have an appetite. In general, reovirus requires no medication, but eyedrops are often prescribed, as well as an antibiotic to protect against secondary bacterial infections. Cats with pneumonitis are slightly more ill. Their eyes may require more treatment but they, too, will usually be only mildly feverish and will continue to eat. Treatment of pneumonitis usually consists of antibiotics and eyedrops or salve. Recovery is usually uneventful. There is a pneumonitis vaccine available through veterinarians. All cats do not need routine pneumonitis prevention, particularly indoor house cats. However, some boarding kennels require proof of vaccination.

Calicivirus infection and rhinotracheitis are more serious. Cats with these diseases run a very high fever and have extremely thick eye and nasal discharges. They may have ulcers or open sores in their mouths. These, in addition to a diminished sense of smell due to a stuffy nose, will cause a cat to become severely anorexic (as we mentioned in Chapter 1, cats' appetites are governed by their sense of smell). This can lead to dehydration, causing a cat to become even sicker as her resistance is lowered.

The rhinotracheitis virus may also cause corneal ulcers. These can be painful and cause squinting. They may lead to permanent corneal scarring. Since this disease is caused by a herpes virus, antiherpes eyedrops may be part of the treatment.

There is a syndrome of the calicivirus called the "limping kitten syndrome," which is characterized by fever and painful, swollen joints.

Left untreated, both calicivirus and rhinotracheitis can be fatal, especially in young kittens. These diseases are much more serious than the "common cold." Older animals will require support and medication for some time, including force-feeding and antibiotics. The likelihood of their survival is good, with proper treatment.

Feline Panleukopenia (also called Feline Distemper)

Panleukopenia is a serious viral disease of cats. This virus is highly contagious and is easily transmitted from cat to cat. It can also be carried by humans on their hands, feet, or clothing. This virus also persists in the environment and is difficult to kill with disinfectants. A dilute bleach solution (one part bleach to nine parts water) is the most effective disinfectant.

Panleukopenia is more common in kittens, prior to vaccination, and those with poor immune systems, although it can occur in adult cats if their immunity fails and they are exposed to an especially virulent strain of the disease. A kitten or cat with panleukopenia will be very sick. She will have gastrointestinal symptoms, including severe diarrhea, dehydration, high fever, severe depression (see definition, page 101), and vomiting. In addition, her bone marrow will be profoundly depressed, the first sign of which is a severe lowering of the white blood cell count. The word "panleukopenia" means depression of all the different kinds of white blood cells.

The combination of a disruption of these two different body systems will cause serious problems. When a cat's gastrointestinal system is damaged by a viral infection it allows bacterial invasion of the body via the bloodstream. Normally, white blood cells eat (phagocytize) the bacteria as they enter the bloodstream. But if the white blood cells are depressed, the bacterial infection can become systemic, leading to septicemia (bacterial infection of the bloodstream). This is the primary cause of death in cats with untreated panleukopenia, although they would probably eventually die from the dehydration caused by vomiting and diarrhea.

Treatment consists of intravenous fluids to rehydrate the cat and control water balance, some supplemental nourishment, and antibiotics. Adult cats that have prompt treatment usually recover. Young kittens have a high mortality rate from panleukopenia, even with treatment. Routine vaccination against this disease is effective and extremely important. See page 18 for kittens' vaccination schedule, page 19 for adults'.

Fungal Feline Diseases

In addition to ringworm (see below), there are several other feline fungal diseases. Cats, however, are less apt to be infected with a fungal disease than dogs.

Aspergillosis is a fungus that usually attacks the respiratory tract of cats and may infect the nose. It is found in the air, the soil, moldy animal feeds, and decaying hay or vegetable matter. Infected animals may have sneezing, nasal discharge, and/or nose bleeds.

There are four *mycoses,* which are fairly uncommon, but may be serious in a cat. These fungal diseases are usually contracted by inhalation, or possibly through the skin, and then spread to the animal's internal organs or other tissues. The fungi that cause these diseases usually prefer particular environments and, therefore, are limited to specific geographic locations.

Blastomycosis is found in the soil in the north-central states, the Ohio-Mississippi River valleys, and the Mid-Atlantic states.

Histoplasmosis is also a soil fungus. It prefers humid, moist soil, and bat, wild-bird, and especially chicken droppings. Histoplasmosis infection is common in the Midwest and East. It is normally characterized by low fever, lethargy, and cough.

Coccidioidomycosis is found in dry, desert areas where the creosote bush grows (central Texas to California), and can affect both cats and humans, but is not contagious.

Of the mycoses, the most common in cats is *cryptococcosis,* which is found in bird droppings, especially that of pigeons, and in soil contaminated by them. It often attacks the central nervous system. Signs are mostly neurologic, including circling, disorientation, head tilt, seizures, and possible paralysis. Diagnosis is made with specialized tests or biopsy. Treatment is difficult; the disease is not always responsive to antifungal medication because the drugs are difficult to deliver to the central nervous system. While not normally considered a contagious disease, it has been nicknamed "pigeon handlers' disease." Therefore, immune-suppressed people should be careful of cats infected with cryptococcosis.

Parasitic Feline Diseases

Many of the parasitic diseases that plague dogs are uncommon or nonexistent in cats. Ticks, the principle carriers of many canine parasitic diseases, do not usually adhere to cats, or are immediately removed by grooming. Therefore, diseases such as Ehrlichiosis, Rocky Mountain Spotted Fever, and Lyme disease are very rare in cats.

Heartworm Disease

Formerly considered only a canine disease, heartworm disease can affect outdoor cats, especially in areas that are heavily infested with mosquitoes. The disease is carried by mosquitoes, which bite an infected animal, ingest immature worm larvae, and then deposit the immature worm larvae into another, uninfected animal's skin and bloodstream. The infective larvae migrate into a cat's heart and lungs, after they develop, where they can grow to enormous lengths and, if left untreated, will eventually cause severe heart and lung damage.

In general, cats with heartworms display fewer symptoms than dogs with the disease.

Therefore, the disease often goes unnoticed in cats. Symptoms may include breathing difficulty, listlessness, coughing, loss of appetite, and surprisingly, vomiting. Treatment of cats with heartworms is extremely dangerous and requires hospitalization and vigilant monitoring.

The best protection for a cat that is likely to be exposed to a number of mosquitoes is the same preventive oral medication used for dogs. If heartworms are a serious problem in the cat's environment, the owner should discuss heartworm prevention for cats with a veterinarian.

Diseases That Cats Can Transmit to People (Zoonotic Diseases)

Although most feline diseases are what are called "species specific," that is, confined only to cats, there are some feline diseases that can be transmitted to people. Rabies, covered above, is the most dangerous. Generally speaking, the best protection against contagion is preventive immunization.

The other important step owners can take to prevent contagion is to pay strict attention to hygiene. Children in particular should be taught to automatically wash their hands after any contact with a cat or her waste, especially before eating, and if they have been playing in an area where cats may deposit waste—sandboxes are particularly attractive to cats. A cat that shares a bed with a person should be kept free from external and internal parasites. Immunocompromised pet owners need to be especially careful to avoid opportunistic zoonotic infections and should discuss ways to prevent transmission with both their veterinarians and personal doctors.

Some of the most common zoonotic diseases associated with cats are:

Cat Scratch Disease (Cat Scratch Fever)

The organism that causes cat scratch disease is a *bacterium* called *Bartonella henselae*. It is a very rare disease but can be transmitted to people by a scratch, bite, and probably by the bite of an infected cat flea. Cats that transmit the disease are usually in good health. It is a disease that is seen worldwide and most commonly affects children and immune-suppressed people. Occasionally an infected cat will become ill and exhibit swollen lymph nodes and fever.

Signs of the disease in people are tender, swollen lymph nodes and possible fever. The disease is usually treated with antibiotics. The best prevention against cat scratch disease is to maintain very good flea control. Fleas appear to be the most common mode of transmission among cats and possibly to people, too.

Toxoplasmosis

Toxoplasmosis is caused by a *protozoan organism*. It can be spread to people via infected cat feces, contaminated soil or litter, or by eating contaminated or rare meat. The most important concern about this disease is for pregnant women; a fetus infected with toxoplasmosis may develop serious problems. Pregnant women should not handle cat feces, soiled litter, or the sand in sandboxes, and should be sure to wash their hands after gardening or any other contact with soil that could be contaminated. They should also avoid raw meat. The same precautions apply to immunosuppressed individuals. Even though cats are the only species that can pass toxoplasma organisms in their stools, all mammals can be infected. Toxoplasmosis should not be the cause of cat hysteria. It is a rather uncommon problem and even infected cats shed infective oocysts for only a short period.

5

Most people are probably infected by eating raw or undercooked meat and not by contact with cats. Proper litter box cleaning and simple hygiene will normally prevent toxoplasma problems.

A cat can get toxoplasmosis from another, infected cat's fecal matter, infected soil that can get on her feet and be licked off when grooming, or from eating infected raw meat or prey such as rodents. An infected cat may have lesions on her lungs, liver, gastrointestinal tract, and brain. The symptoms will vary depending on the organs infected. The brain is commonly affected, seizures and other neurologic signs may develop. Nonapparent infection can also occur in cats.

Ringworm

Ringworm is a *fungal* skin disease to which cats, dogs, and humans, especially children, are highly susceptible. Children should not be allowed to touch a cat suspected of having the disease. It is primarily spread by direct contact, although spores can be airborne. A cat may carry ringworm fungus without symptoms and act as a source of infection to other pets and people. These "carrier" cats may develop lesions when they are stressed or diseased. However, even after the lesions clear, they main remain infected.

Ringworm lesions on cats are usually patchy, somewhat round, hairless areas, which can also be scaly. These types of lesions should be investigated by a veterinarian. Diagnosis is usually made by fungal culture of infected hairs or examination of infected hairs under a microscope. Some ringworm lesions fluoresce under an ultraviolet light. Treatment in cats often involves complete shaving of the hair (carefully collecting all the hair in a plastic bag) and treatment with

dips and possibly oral medication. The most common oral medicine for ringworm is griseofulvin. This medicine is toxic to and may even kill some cats.

Parasites

Fleas can and will go from cats to humans given the opportunity. To prevent this from happening, proper treatment of an affected cat and her environment is necessary. See Chapter 2, page 30 for more about this.

As we stated in Chapter 2, page 16, roundworms (toxocara) can infect people (the condition is known as toxocariasis) and owners must be sure to eradicate roundworms, following a veterinarian's instructions.

CONTAGIOUS AND INFECTIOUS FELINE DISEASES

Care of an Injured or Sick Cat

When a pet cat is injured an owner often must make some immediate decisions about what to do and how to do it. If a cat is ill or recuperating from surgery or injury, the owner must be prepared to look after him and tend to his needs, which may include giving medications and caring for bandages. In the case of a chronic illness such as diabetes mellitus or other long-term problem, an owner may be called on to medicate a cat for the rest of the animal's life. In this chapter we will include a brief rundown of some of the more commonly occurring emergency and recuperative situations and how to deal with them.

Emergency First Aid Steps

Most injuries and serious illnesses require immediate veterinary care as we pointed out in Chapter 4. It is a waste of precious time for an owner to attempt first aid steps that may do more harm than good in the end. However, there are certainly situations in which something must be done to make a cat more comfortable and, perhaps, to save his life, especially in the case of traumatic injury. An owner must attempt to stop serious bleeding, and an injured cat must be transported to the veterinary office or emergency clinic in a way that will do him no further harm.

Handle With Care!

A severely injured cat is likely to be in pain and will also be badly frightened. An owner should realize that the first thing an injured cat will try to do is run away and hide, so she must be prepared to secure the cat right away. If he is too badly injured to run off, he may strike out at anyone, even his owner, when he is approached or touched. Anyone attempting to minister to an injured cat should protect her arms and hands as well as possible, and should avoid putting her face near the cat's.

As we mentioned in Chapter 2, some sort of secure carrying case should be a standard piece of equipment for all cats. If there is no carrying case available to put an injured cat in, the best way to secure the cat and prevent being scratched is to wrap him, securely but gently, in a towel, small blanket, sweater, or other piece of clothing. Wrap his body and legs, leaving his head out. He can then be placed in a carton or box, or someone's lap, and held while being transported to the veterinarian. It is best to

Signs of Pain

Cats handle pain with varying degrees of stoicism, just as all animals do. Many cats are fearful of strange people and unfamiliar experiences. Sometimes the very fact of going to a veterinarian's office and perhaps having even a minor procedure performed will cause a cat to react as if he is in pain when he returns home.

A cat that is in slight pain after minor surgery, for instance, will definitely want to be left alone to "sleep it off," often in a dark, hard-to-get-at area of his own choosing, such as way underneath a bed or other heavy piece of furniture. As long as an owner knows the cat is all right, she can leave him alone up to twenty-four hours until he is ready to come out. She should be sure to leave a bowl of fresh water and a litter tray within easy reach and keep children and other pets out of the room. If a cat "hides out" for longer than a day, it may be necessary to get him out, check him over, and possibly force-feed him (see page 74) to help him on the road to recovery.

A cat that hurts badly may not want to move. He will be anorectic, his pupils will be dilated, he will pant rapidly, and cry out or yowl in pain. He should not be allowed to hide, because he obviously needs immediate veterinary help. Cats in pain often bite, so it is important for an owner to protect herself by wearing gloves and long sleeves if she is going to handle a badly hurting cat.

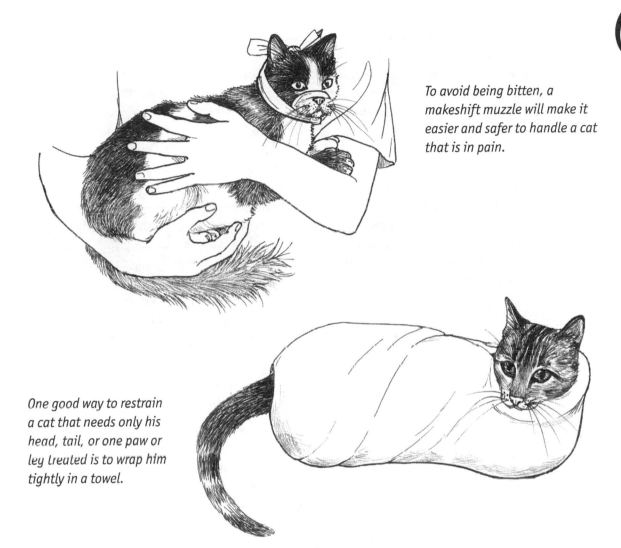

To avoid being bitten, a makeshift muzzle will make it easier and safer to handle a cat that is in pain.

One good way to restrain a cat that needs only his head, tail, or one paw or leg treated is to wrap him tightly in a towel.

engage a helper's assistance, because even a badly injured cat may be able to work his way out of a wrap and injure himself further.

Stopping Bleeding

We discussed the use of a *pressure bandage,* and how to apply one, in Chapter 4, page 56. In the case of spurting, arterial bleeding it may be necessary to apply manual pressure with a clean cloth or bandage placed on top of the wound to stop the flow of blood; then a pressure bandage can be applied. As we stated in Chapter 4, we do not advocate the use of tourniquets because they can easily cause permanent limb or extremity damage.

Resuscitation

If a cat is not breathing (apnea), or his heart is not beating (this can be readily ascertained by feeling the chest area for a heartbeat), immediate action must be taken to avoid brain damage. If the cause is electrocution from biting a plugged-in electric wire, be sure the wire is unplugged before touching the cat. It is rare for a cat to drown, but cats can stop breathing due to smoke inhalation or a chest wound.

It is important to note here that, in a case of full-blown cardiac arrest, even the best-equipped intensive care facilities in major veterinary hospitals with expert staff have only a 4 percent rate of success in resuscitating cats. Therefore, the chances of an owner being able to successfully resuscitate a cat with cardiac arrest are very slim. Most owners, however, feel they must try.

ARTIFICIAL RESPIRATION

The easiest way to perform artificial respiration to start a cat breathing again is by *mouth-to-nose resuscitation.* The cat's mouth should be sealed tightly closed using two hands, then the person's mouth should be placed firmly around the cat's nose. With gentle blowing into the nose for several seconds eight to ten times per minute, the cat may be encouraged to breathe on his own. Once the cat has begun to breathe he should be taken to the veterinarian right away.

CARDIOPULMONARY RESUSCITATION (CPR)

If a cat has stopped breathing *and* his heart is not beating, he may be helped by CPR, a combination of heart massage and artificial respiration. As we pointed out above, however, this procedure is hardly ever successful.

The cat should be put on his side on a hard surface. His airways should be cleared by pulling out his tongue and checking inside his mouth and throat before beginning. First, mouth-to-nose resuscitation should be performed. If there is still no heartbeat, heart massage can be per-

formed. A cat's heart is located just behind his front legs. With gentle pressure, the heel of a hand should compress the cat's chest and then release it in a regular rhythm. This should be repeated about six to ten times, then mouth-to-nose resuscitation repeated. If no pulse is felt, the process may be repeated, but if no positive results are seen after approximately ten minutes, the process is probably in vain. The best course to take is to have someone try to obtain veterinary help, or drive to the veterinarian with the cat while the resuscitation effort is under way. As an alternative to laying a cat down and using the heel of the hand, a person can grasp a cat's chest behind the front legs with the thumb on one side and finger on the other side. The chest can be compressed rhythmically during transportation.

Home Care of a Sick or Recuperating Cat

Inexperienced cat owners, in particular, are often very concerned about their ability to take care of or medicate a sick or recuperating cat. Some cats are extremely difficult to medicate, and even the best-natured cat requiring regular medication will quickly learn to run off and hide as soon as he sees or smells the medicine. An owner will soon know if this is the case with a particular cat and should confine the cat in one room (preferably one with few pieces of large furniture to get under, such as a kitchen or bathroom) well before the medication needs to be given.

If a cat simply cannot be medicated at home, the veterinarian may be able to help. Sometimes, a different form of medicine may be easier for an owner to use, or a cat may have to be taken to the doctor's office in order to be medicated.

6

Restraints and Tricks

It is always easier to medicate or treat a cat when he is up on a counter or tabletop. It is also preferable to have a helper who can stand behind the animal and hold him while he is being treated. To give oral medication or treat a cat's head or mouth, the helper can hold the cat in her arms, grasping his front legs so he cannot scratch.

Many cats become very frightened when they are restrained too firmly. A good-natured cat, placed on a counter or tabletop, may only require gentle holding while he is medicated.

If a procedure is painful or unpleasant, or if a cat is very panicky or aggressive, more serious restraint may be needed. A cat that is frightened or aggressive will probably strike out, so owner and helper should protect their arms and hands before attempting treatment or medication. One good way to restrain a cat that needs only his head or one paw or leg treated is to wrap his whole body in a towel. Gently shaking a cat by the loose skin at the back of his neck will often distract him sufficiently to perform a quick procedure on his body. Another way to keep a cat quiet for an examination or brief procedure is to have a helper stretch the cat out to his full length on his side on a counter or tabletop by holding his neck and back legs.

If it is still impossible for an owner to medicate or treat a cat at home, he may have to be hospitalized and tranquilized for treatment.

A cat that immediately tries to lick off any ointment or salve, chew off a bandage, or scratch his head or ears, for instance, may need to wear an *Elizabethan collar* for a while. This is a soft plastic cone, available from a veterinarian, that ties or snaps around the animal's neck behind his ears and extends beyond the tip of his nose so that he cannot get his mouth to any part of his body or scratch any part of his head or ears (see illustration, page 76). Cats hate these devices but they are sometimes necessary on a temporary basis. The collar must be removed at intervals, under strict supervision in a closed room, to allow the cat to groom himself, eat, and drink. Do not allow the cat to escape. It will be very difficult to locate and recollar him if you do!

General Daily Care of a Sick Cat

A cat that is sick or recuperating from an operation or accident is in a somewhat fragile condition. That is, he is apt to be more sensitive to extremes of temperature, and more bothered by loud noise and commotion. Just as with a human patient, a cat that doesn't feel well should be kept warm and protected from roughhousing children and other pets. Many cats really want to be left alone when they are not well; others crave loving attention from their owners, or from one special owner. An owner should take her cue from her pet in this regard.

Most cats have one or more favorite sleeping places and should be allowed to have the run of the house so they can choose where to sleep. An owner must be sure the cat is warm enough wherever he sleeps; an extra blanket, or even a heat lamp above the cat's sleeping area, may be needed if the house is cool. If a cat persists in hiding underneath a heavy piece of furniture, he must be removed from time to time, forcibly if necessary, so he can be given food and fluids. If a sick or recuperating cat is unable or unwilling to venture out of a room in the house, he must have a litter tray, food, and water nearby.

An owner may be asked by the veterinarian to *take the cat's temperature* on a regular basis. The veterinarian should demonstrate how to do this, but basically, a helper is recommended. Cats' anal-rectal muscles are very strong and it may be difficult to slip a thermometer in. The cat should be placed on a counter or tabletop. A rectal thermometer lubricated with vaseline or mineral oil should be used, shaken down, and inserted until only about one inch is visible. It should remain in place for one minute. A normal temperature for a cat is about 100 to 102.5 degrees Fahrenheit.

Cats often become *anorexic* when they are ill. This is especially true if their sense of smell has been affected. Sometimes, very strong-smelling fishy food will encourage a cat to begin to eat again. If this doesn't work it may be necessary to *force-feed* a cat. Nutrients in paste form, such as strained baby food that does not contain onion powder, can be placed on a fingertip and wiped directly onto the roof of a cat's mouth. Alternately, liquid nutrients can be placed in a large dropper or syringe, available from a veterinarian or pharmacist. Tilting the cat's head

upward, pull his cheek out gently to form a funnellike opening into which the liquid can be squeezed. It will trickle into the animal's mouth through his teeth. Water should be given in the same manner.

Medicating a Cat

As we mentioned above, medicating even the best-tempered cat can be very difficult, even for experienced cat owners. Three basic rules apply for successfully giving oral medication to a cat: learn to anticipate a cat's attempts to escape; get help when needed; stay calm; and be patient. Because cats are such good escape artists and seem to be able to know way in advance when a medication is going to be given, the primary rule is to confine a cat well ahead of time.

Liquid medicine is the easiest to administer to many cats. As with forcing liquids above, hold the cat close to the body and tilt the cat's head back. Hold the cat's mouth closed and insert the dropper or syringe tip in the side of the mouth in the cheek pouch. Administer the medicine in this pouch and it will run through the teeth into the mouth. If the mouth is held closed it will make it difficult for the cat to spit out the medicine. Unfortunately, many liquid medicines are elixirs (alcohol-based), which cats do not like. Others are flavored for humans, especially children, and have fruit flavors

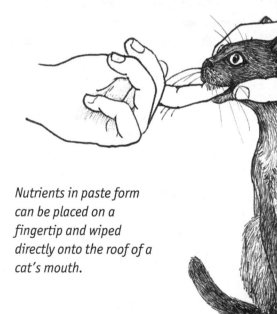

Nutrients in paste form can be placed on a fingertip and wiped directly onto the roof of a cat's mouth.

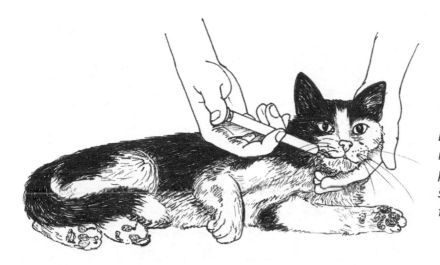

Liquid nutrients or medicine can be placed in a large syringe and squeezed into a cat's mouth.

that cat palates do not appreciate. Some pharmacies will compound liquid medicines in cat-friendly flavors such as fish or chicken.

Pills and capsules cannot be hidden in food for cats as they can for dogs; cats will simply spit them out. Pilling a cat usually requires a second person to hold the cat from behind to keep him from backing up. With some cats, wrapping them up in a blanket or towel can replace the helper. The person administering the pill should grab the cat's head with the palm of the hand over the nose, thumb on one side of the upper jaw and index finger on the other side (see illustration, right). Tilt the cat's head back and open the mouth with the other hand by pressing down on the lower jaw as the top jaw is squeezed with the first hand. The pill is then inserted over the tongue and toward the back of the throat (see illustration, above right). It should be given a quick push over the hump of the tongue and the mouth quickly closed. Then blow gently on the cat's face and

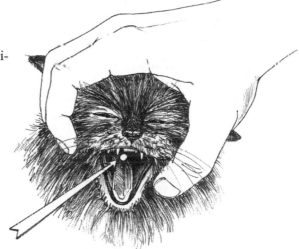

Pilling a cat. Note where the pill should be placed.

massage his throat, which will encourage him to swallow. This difficult process does improve with practice.

Eye medicine comes in two basic forms, liquid drops and ointment. In either case, it is important not to poke or scratch the cornea with

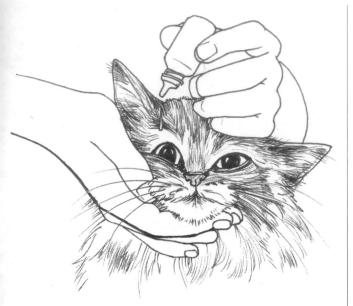

When applying drops be very careful not to poke the cat in the eye. Rest your hand on top of the animal's head to steady it.

the applicator tip. The cat must be held still (helper or blanket wrap) and the medicine should be placed in the corner of the eye nearest the nose. This is where the third eyelid is and this organ helps protect the cornea from the applicator tip. It also helps to rest the hand holding the applicator on the top of the cat's head to steady it (see illustration, above). The medicine can then be placed in the lower eyelid. After applying the medicine, close the eyelids so the medicine will be distributed over the entire eye.

Ear medicine is usually fairly easy to apply to a cat, unless his ears are very sore or tender. It also comes in liquid or ointment form. Hold the cat's head steady with one hand, place the applicator directly into the ear canal, and squeeze. It is not necessary to stick the tip all the way into the ear. Then massage the area beneath the ear to spread the medicine into the ear canal, which runs down the side of a cat's head.

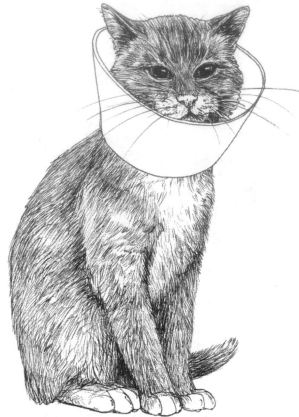

An Elizabethan collar will prevent a cat from scratching his head or ears, licking ointment or salve off his body, or chewing a bandage. The collar must be removed at intervals, under strict supervision, to allow the cat to eat and drink.

Skin ointments and salves are easy to apply. The trick is to keep a cat from immediately licking them off. Sometimes a distraction such as a delicious meal, favorite toy, or gentle brushing may distract the cat long enough for the medicine to work (approximately ten to fifteen minutes). If a cat cannot be distracted and it is very important for the medication to remain on his skin, an Elizabethan collar (see page 73 and illustration, above) may be necessary, especially at night when no one is watching the cat.

If a cat requires *injections* at home, the veterinarian will demonstrate how to give them.

Sometimes *medicated baths* are prescribed, especially for skin conditions. Follow the instructions for bathing a cat in Chapter 2, page 30.

If it is impossible for an owner to treat a cat at home, the cat may need to be hospitalized.

Casts and Bandages

Casts and bandages are usually left alone between veterinary visits. The hardest job for an owner is to keep them dry and as clean as possible, especially if a cat is allowed outdoors. It is usually not a good idea to allow a cat free range outdoors if he is wearing a cast or large bandage because his mobility will be affected and he will be unable to escape from dogs or other cats.

If a cat persistently chews or scratches a bandage or cast, or constantly licks the area around it, it may be necessary to use an Elizabethan collar (left) to prevent soreness and infection from developing. If an owner notices a bad smell or any swelling, irritation, or redness around a cast or bandage or in any part of a bandaged limb, such as a paw, the veterinarian should be contacted immediately. Most bandages or casts will leave toes exposed at the bottom of the bandage. An owner should check the toes often (several times a day) to see if the toes are swollen. Any swelling of the toes should be checked by a veterinarian; it usually indicates a bandage or cast that is too tight or has slipped, interfering with circulation to the lower limb.

Part Three

More Than 130

of the Most Commonly Seen

Feline Signs / Symptoms

of Illness, and

How to Interpret Them

Index of More Than 130 Signs/ Symptoms *

*Bold entries are alphabetically listed as headings in "More Than 130 of the Most Commonly Seen Feline Signs/Symptoms of Illness, and How to Interpret Them," pp. 93–141.

More Than 130 of the

Most Commonly Seen

Feline Signs/Symptoms

of Illness, and

How to Interpret Them

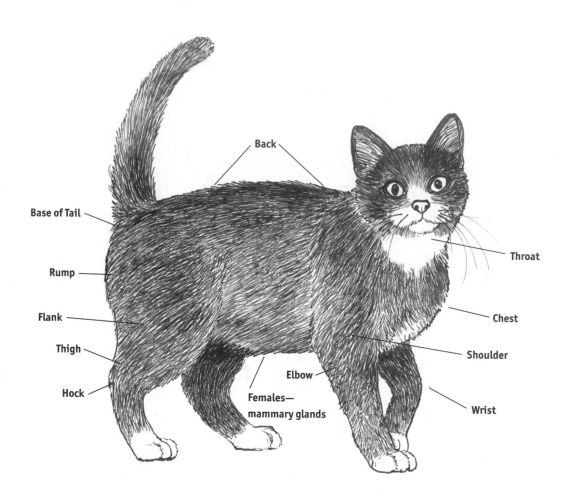

Side View of a Cat

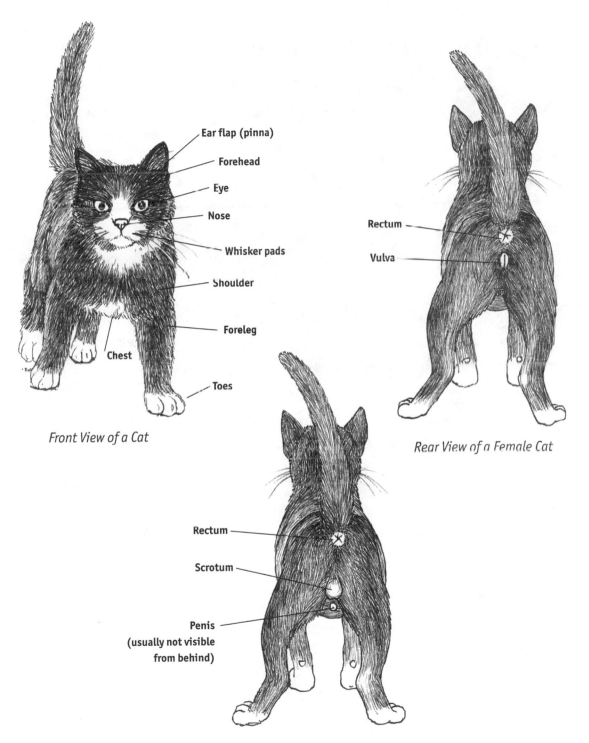

Ear flap (pinna)

Forehead

Eye

Nose

Whisker pads

Shoulder

Foreleg

Chest

Toes

Front View of a Cat

Rectum

Vulva

Rear View of a Female Cat

Rectum

Scrotum

Penis
(usually not visible
from behind)

Rear View of an Unneutered Male Cat

Abdominal Distension

Any change in the shape or size of a cat's abdomen should be carefully assessed. The term "abdominal distension" implies that the abdomen slowly enlarges so that there are clearly bulges when the cat is viewed from the top. From the side, it may have what most people refer to as a potbellied appearance. A cat's stomach may appear larger than normal due to pregnancy, excess fat accumulation either in the abdomen itself or underneath the surrounding skin, an accumulation of gas or fluid in the stomach or intestines, an infection that causes swelling, an obstruction of the urinary tract, or a growth or enlargement of the liver or spleen.

Sign/Symptom	Observations	Associated Signs	Possible Condition	Action to Take
Chronic abdominal distension	Cat feels fine (Note: A cat should never be starved or have her calorie intake drastically reduced. Weight loss should always be gradual. Begin by reducing intake by 10 to 20 percent.)	None	Obesity	Consult veterinarian for dietary changes. Low-calorie diet; less food.
Chronic abdominal distension	Cat is not having bowel movements.	Eventually becomes anorexic. Vomiting. Dehydration.	Obstipation (impaction of colon with feces, also called megacolon).	Take to veterinarian for treatment (deobstipation), stool softeners, possible surgery if advanced.
Progressive abdominal distension over past two months	Intact female cat	Possible mammary gland enlargement	Pregnancy	See veterinarian for confirmation and instructions.
Abdominal distension	Intact female cat. Not feeling well.	Possibly mucoid or bloody vaginal discharge. Fever.	Pyometra (uterine infection) (see p. 53; see also Box, below)	See veterinarian for tests, X rays, surgery.

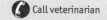

Home care; first aid   Call veterinarian   Call veterinarian; make appointment within 24 hours

Sign/Symptom	Observations	Associated Signs	Possible Condition	Action to Take
Slowly increasing abdominal distension	Possibly more noticeable on one side. May not be feeling well. May have depressed appetite.	Weight loss. Possible vomiting, diarrhea, jaundice (see Glossary).	Abdominal mass in the liver, spleen, kidney, intestine	See veterinarian for tests, X rays, possible ultrasound, possible surgery.
Progressive abdominal distension	Abdomen is soft, symetrically shaped	May have muscle loss, lethargy, depressed appetite. Possible fever (see pp. 73–74 for how to take a cat's temperature).	Fluid in abdomen, caused by heart disease (see p. 52), FIP (see pp. 60–61), peritonitis (see Glossary). Cancer. Liver failure.	See veterinarian for tests, X rays
Acute abdominal distension	Recent history of trauma	Depressed. Anorectic. Possible fever. Possibly pale mucous membranes (see "Shock," p. 55).	Ruptured bladder. If pale = hemorrhage. If fever = peritonitis (see Glossary).	Go to emergency clinic for tests and possible surgery.
Acute abdominal distension	Respiratory distress, dyspnea (difficulty breathing)	Depression. Anorexia.	Stomach enlargement due to swallowed air.	Go to emergency clinic for oxygen, possible X rays.
Rapid abdominal distension	Weak. Lethargic.	Pale mucous membranes (see "Shock," p. 55) Possible hypothermia (low body temperature).	Anemia due to bleeding into abdomen (trauma, tumor, rat poison [see "Poisoning," pp. 50–51; see also Appendix A, p. 145])	Go to emergency clinic for tests, medication, possible surgery.

A

B
D
O
M
I
N
A
L

D
I
S
T
E
N
S
I
O
N

Pyometra*

A pyometra is a uterine infection, which is a very common condition in old, unspayed female cats. It is one of the many reasons why female cats should be spayed. In a closed pyometra, the pus builds up and the uterus distends like a sausage. In a draining pyometra, pus clearly discharges from the vulva. Surgical removal of the uterus is the correct treatment.

*See also p. 53.

Call veterinarian; make appointment immediately   Life-threatening condition; go *immediately* to veterinarian or emergency clinic

Appetite, Abnormal

Any alteration in the way a cat approaches her food should not be overlooked. A cat that has always been finicky will often decide to skip a meal or two. If the cat is acting fine, there is no need for concern. However, if a cat stops eating or obviously eats less and is not acting well at the same time, it is the sign of a problem. Conversely, a cat that suddenly eats a lot more than usual may have a medical problem.

A completely different type of abnormal appetite that some cats exhibit is a particular form of pica (the eating of inappropriate things), wool eating (or wool sucking).

Sign/Symptom	Observations	Associated Signs	Possible Condition	Action to Take
Increase in appetite	Crying for food	Weight increase	Spoiled cat, or cat enjoying food too much. Diet too palatable.	✚ Feed less. Feed lower-calorie food.
	(Note: Do not feed the cat when she cries; this obviously rewards the behavior.)			
Increase in appetite	May develop large abdomen and severe hair loss.	Increased thirst and urination	Diabetes mellitus secondary to Cushing's syndrome, fairly rare in cats (see Glossary)	🐾 See veterinarian for tests.
Increase in appetite	Cannot get enough food. Losing weight.	Increased thirst and urination	Diabetes mellitus (see Glossary)	🐾 See veterinarian for tests and treatment options. Bring urine sample if possible.
Increase in appetite	Losing weight	Diarrhea and/or vomiting	Not absorbing nutrients due to diarrhea; parasites; IBD— inflammatory bowel disease (see Glossary); hyperthyroidism; exocrine pancreatic insufficiency (EPI).	🐾 See veterinarian for tests, treatment.

✚ Home care; first aid   🐾 Call veterinarian   🐾 Call veterinarian; make appointment within 24 hours

Sign/Symptom	Observations	Associated Signs	Possible Condition	Action to Take
Increase in appetite	Older cat. Losing weight. May be hyperactive.	Possible diarrhea, vomiting	Hyperthyroidism (thyroid tumor) (see Glossary)	See veterinarian for tests and treatment options.
Decreased appetite	Possibly lethargic	Possible vomiting, diarrhea, drooling, weight loss	Nausea from: intestinal parasites; IBD—inflammatory bowel disease (see Glossary); plant ingestion; infection; urinary obstruction; cancer; kidney/liver disease; intestinal foreign body; obstipation (see Glossary).	See veterinarian for tests and possible medication.
Depressed appetite	Lethargic, feels warm (see pp. 73–74 for how to take a cat's temperature)	None	Fever due to: infection (abscess; upper respiratory infection, or URI—see pp. 63–64; leukemia (see pp. 61–62); FIV (see p. 61); cancer, immune-mediated disease.	See veterinarian for tests, medication. *Do not give aspirin, acetaminophen, ibuprofin, or any other over-the-counter medicine to cats.*
Depressed appetite	Lethargic	Pale mucous membranes	Anemia due to: blood loss; FeLV (see pp. 61–62); cancer; kidney disease; immune-mediated disease; drug ingestion; rat poison (see "Poisoning," pp. 50–51, and p. 57; see also Appendix A, p. 145)	Go to emergency clinic for tests, possible transfusion.

 Call veterinarian; make appointment immediately   Life-threatening condition; go *immediately* to veterinarian or emergency clinic

Sign/Symptom	Observations	Associated Signs	Possible Condition	Action to Take
Depressed appetite	Lethargy. Difficulty breathing.	Possible cough	Cardiac disease (see "Cardiovascular Emergencies," p. 52). Lung cancer. Pneumonia. Fluid in lungs or chest cavity.	Go to emergency clinic for X rays, medication, possible ultrasound.
Eats fabric, especially wool	Usually Siamese cats	May lead to vomiting, intestinal obstruction	Wool eater	Put all wool away. See veterinarian for behavior-modifying medication. (Note: This is thought to be a form of compulsive behavior.)

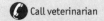
Home care; first aid   Call veterinarian   Call veterinarian; make appointment within 24 hours

Depression/Lethargy

When a cat is *depressed,* he will show little interest in things that normally excite him, such as playing, being petted, and interacting with his owners and other pets. He may hide under furniture, etc. *Lethargy* manifests itself by a lack of activity. This may be difficult to assess in a cat, especially an older animal, because cats normally sleep up to eighteen hours a day. However, when an owner knows her pet, it is usually not difficult to tell when he just is not feeling well. Depression and lethargy are not normal, but are nonspecific signs of an underlying medical problem. As most serious diseases progress, a cat will eventually become depressed, stop eating and drinking, and become progressively more depressed.

Sign/Symptom	Observations	Associated Signs	Possible Condition	Action to Take
Depression/lethargy	Feels warm. Temperature is more than 103 degrees at rest. (See pp. 73–74 for how to take a cat's temperature.)	Anorexia	Fever, any infection, cancer. Rarely, immune-mediated disease.	See veterinarian for confirmation, possible tests, and medication.
Depression/lethargy	Reluctance to walk	Pain if picked up	Pain due to: orthopedic cause; abscess; bladder obstruction; peritonitis	See veterinarian for examination.
Depression/lethargy	Possible anorexia	Possible cough. Difficulty breathing (dyspnea). Purple/blue tongue (cyanosis)	Cardiac disease (see p. 52). Lung disease (cancer, asthma, pneumonia). Fluid in chest cavity (pleural effusion) due to: cancer; cardiac problems; chylothorax (see Glossary); pyothorax (see Glossary). Pneumothorax (from trauma).	Go to emergency clinic for tests, X rays.

 Call veterinarian; make appointment immediately   Life-threatening condition; go *immediately* to veterinarian or emergency clinic

Sign/Symptom	Observations	Associated Signs	Possible Condition	Action to Take
Depression/lethargy	Anorexia	Pale mucous membranes	Anemia, due to: FeLV (see pp. 61–62); FIV (see p. 61); drugs or rat poison (see pp. 50–51); blood loss; immune-mediated disease; cancer; kidney disease	Go to emergency clinic for tests, possible transfusion.
Depression/lethargy	Diabetic cat being treated with insulin.	Possible collapse, coma, seizures	Hypoglycemia secondary to insulin overdose or inadequate food intake	See veterinarian, or go to emergency clinic if seizures, coma, or collapse
Depression/lethargy	Usually older cat. Anorexia, weight loss.	Increased thirst, bad breath, possible anemia	Kidney disease— a tumor, infection, acute or chronic nephritis (inflammation of the kidney); diabetes mellitus	See veterinarian for tests.
Depression/lethargy	Male cat. Straining to urinate. Possibly painful if picked up.	Anorexia. Possible vomiting.	Urinary tract obstruction. (FLUTD [FUS]—see "Urinary Emergencies," p. 54)	Go to emergency clinic for catheterization, fluids, possible X rays.
Depression/lethargy	Anorexia. Possible weight loss.	Vomiting. Possible diarrhea.	Gastroenteritis (irritated stomach or intestines) due to: infection; foreign body ingestion (e.g., string, ribbon, plants, drugs); cancer; liver/kidney disease; pancreatitis (inflammation of the pancreas)	See veterinarian for tests, medication, possible fluids, and X rays.

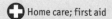 Home care; first aid   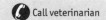 Call veterinarian   Call veterinarian; make appointment within 24 hours

Sign/Symptom	Observations	Associated Signs	Possible Condition	Action to Take
Depression/lethargy	Anorexia	Jaundice (see Glossary). Possible vomiting.	Liver disease (tumor, inflammation, fatty infiltration, FIP [see pp. 60–61]; peritonitis)	🐾 See veterinarian for tests, possible X rays.
Depression/lethargy, progressive	May not recognize people or interact with other pets	Possibly blind. Possible seizures. Possible weakness. Possible personality changes.	Brain lesion (brain tumor; vascular [blood vessel] accident; trauma; rabies [see p. 63]; encephalitis [see Glossary]; FeLV [see pp. 61–62]); FIP (see pp. 60–61); toxoplasmosis (see pp. 66–67); lead poisoning (see p. 146)	🐾 See veterinarian for tests, possible MRI (see Glossary), possible CAT scan (see Glossary). ✚ If seizures, go to emergency clinic.

D
E
P
R
E
S
S
I
O
N
/
L
E
T
H
A
R
G
Y

🐾 Call veterinarian; make appointment immediately   ✚ Life-threatening condition; go *immediately* to veterinarian or emergency clinic

Diarrhea

Cats are more apt to have chronic rather than acute diarrhea. As a rule, dietary indiscretion is less apt to be a factor with cats than it is in dogs. In order for a veterinarian to diagnose and treat diarrhea in a cat, it is important for an owner to supply information that will determine whether the problem is arising in the small or large intestine. A large volume of episodic watery stool usually implies small-intestinal problems. Small, frequent or continual stools containing small amounts of mucus, sometimes blood, and often accompanied with straining point toward a problem with the colon or large intestine. The stomach is often also involved when a cat is suffering from diarrhea, causing nausea or vomiting.

Weight loss is an important indicator of the seriousness of diarrhea in cats. As a rule, chronic, progressive diarrhea will lead to weight loss and will be more difficult to cure.

A few episodes of diarrhea in an otherwise healthy cat may be safely treated with home care (see Box, p. 106). However, if a cat is lethargic, or other signs persist, veterinary assessment and treatment is called for.

Sign/Symptom	Observations	Associated Signs	Possible Condition	Action to Take
Diarrhea, acute, one to several times	Cat feels all right. Watery or mucoid.	Possible vomiting	Dietary indiscretion. Diet change. Intestinal parasites. Bacterial or viral disease. Drug-induced.	✚ Home treatment of routine diarrhea or vomiting (see Box, p. 106). 📞 If persists more than twenty-four hours, see veterinarian. Bring stool sample.

✚ Home care; first aid   📞 Call veterinarian   📞24 Call veterinarian; make appointment within 24 hours

Sign/Symptom	Observations	Associated Signs	Possible Condition	Action to Take
Chronic, watery diarrhea	Slow weight loss or no weight loss	Vomiting	Inflammatory bowel disease (IBD—see Glossary, usually old cat). Parasite infestation. Food allergy. Dietary indiscretion. Infection. Drug-induced condition (see p. 50).	See veterinarian for tests, possible biopsy. Bring stool sample.
Chronic, watery diarrhea	Weight loss	Possible vomiting	Inflammatory bowel disease (IBD—see Glossary). Intestinal cancer. Fungal infection. Hyperthyroidism (see Glossary). Bacterial overgrowth in intestine.	See veterinarian for medication, tests, possible biopsy. Bring stool sample.
Black, tarry stool	Feces are dark black in color.	Possible vomiting. Possible pale mucous membranes.	Upper gastrointestinal bleeding, due to stomach tumor, stomach ulcer, small intestinal tumor	See veterinarian as soon as possible for tests, X rays, possible surgery, possible blood transfusion.
Chronic, mucoid diarrhea	Strains to move bowels. Sometimes red blood in stool.	Possible weight loss	Colitis. Dietary indiscretion. Colonic cancer or polyps. Bacterial infection. Parasites. Inflammatory bowel disease (IBD—see Glossary). Dietary allergy. Obstipation (colon impaction).	See veterinarian for tests, possible biopsy. Bring stool sample.

 Call veterinarian; make appointment immediately

 Life-threatening condition; go *immediately* to veterinarian or emergency clinic

Home Treatment of Routine Diarrhea or Vomiting

If a cat is suffering from diarrhea or is vomiting and seems to be in good general health otherwise, the first thing to do is withhold all food for twenty-four hours and restrict water intake to small drinks every few hours.* If a cat is vomiting a great deal, water should be restricted to *very* small amounts. (Withholding *all* water may lead to dehydration.) This allows the cat's digestive system to rest, and prevents the loss of fluids from the body, which might cause dehydration. After the cat has stopped vomiting, give him more sips of water. If it is kept down, somewhat larger amounts of water can then be given gradually. For diarrhea, a coating agent, such as Kaopectate, is sometimes recommended by veterinarians. After twenty-four hours, a small amount of bland food can be offered. Well-cooked white rice mixed with pieces of skinless chicken breast that has been boiled to remove any fat is usually well tolerated and binding. This diet should be given for several days after a bout of diarrhea or vomiting. If vomiting or diarrhea persists, further veterinary evaluation is needed.

*Note: It is dangerous to withhold all food from a kitten, as he may develop hypoglycemia (low blood sugar). If the patient is a young kitten, call the veterinarian for advice.

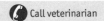

Home care; first aid   Call veterinarian   Call veterinarian; make appointment within 24 hours

Ear Problems

A cat will usually signal her owner when her ears are bothering her by shaking her head or scratching her ears. If she does this, an owner should examine the affected ear for unusual odor or discharge (normally, cats have very little ear wax). He should compare both ears to be sure that the color and texture of the insides are the same. A cat has a long ear canal (see illustration, below) that cannot be easily seen without an otoscope. Therefore, even if an owner sees no abnormality but the cat continues to be uncomfortable, a veterinary assessment is called for.

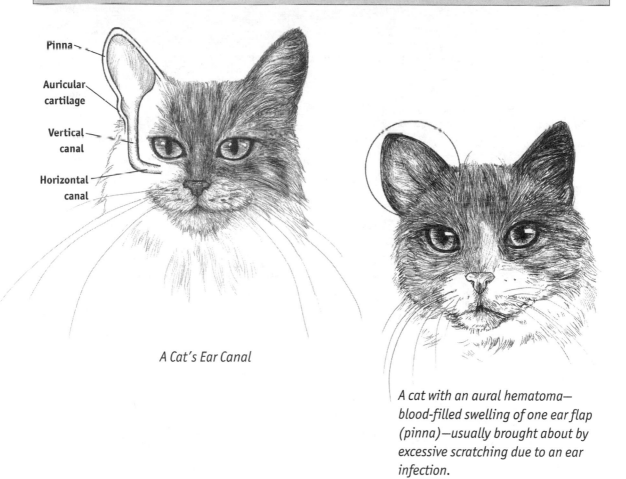

Pinna

Auricular cartilage

Vertical canal

Horizontal canal

A Cat's Ear Canal

A cat with an aural hematoma— blood-filled swelling of one ear flap (pinna)—usually brought about by excessive scratching due to an ear infection.

Call veterinarian; make appointment immediately

Life-threatening condition; go *immediately* to veterinarian or emergency clinic

Sign/Symptom	Observations	Associated Signs	Possible Condition	Action to Take
Shaking head, scratching ears	Usually outdoor cat, or in contact with outdoor cat	Variable amounts of black wax	Ear mites	See veterinarian for diagnosis and medication.
Shaking head, scratching ears	Foul odor from ear	Dark orange or purulent (containing pus) discharge	External ear infection (bacterial or yeast)	See veterinarian for tests, medication.
Swelling of one ear flap (pinna)	Soft, nonpainful swelling	May have external ear infection (see above)	Aural hematoma (blood-filled swelling)	See veterinarian for drainage and to treat underlying problem. Possible surgery.
Swelling of one ear flap (pinna)	Acute onset. Painful. May have been in cat fight.	Possible fever	Abscess	See veterinarian for antibiotics, possible drainage.
Inside of ear and canal has bumpy, often dark appearance	May or may not bother cat	Often has external ear infection, characterized by redness or abnormal discharge.	Polyps	See veterinarian to treat any underlying infection. Possible surgery.
Ears and head very itchy	Scratches and rubs head	Ears and head are red and have scabby lesions	Allergic reaction, often to food. Mange.	See veterinarian for tests, treatment.
Scabby, ulcerated areas along ear edges	Often white or light-colored cat	May have similar lesions elsewhere	Tumor (usually squamous cell carcinoma—see Glossary)	See veterinarian for biopsy, surgery, and to discuss other treatment.
Head tilt	May not want to move. Appetite depressed.	May fall toward side of head tilt. May have external ear infection (see above)	Middle- or inner-ear problem (infection, tumor). Feline vestibular (balance) syndrome.	See veterinarian for X rays, tests.

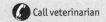 Home care; first aid   Call veterinarian   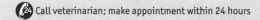 Call veterinarian; make appointment within 24 hours

Eye Disorders

It is often very difficult for an owner to evaluate a cat's eyes. In addition, without the correct terminology, it is hard for her to describe her observations to a veterinarian. If a cat's eyes simply do not look right, it may be due to an internal problem, and a veterinarian should be consulted as soon as possible.

Most veterinarians are familiar with commonly seen feline ocular disorders, and are capable of treating them. There have been many advancements in the treatment of the more complex and obscure eye diseases, however. Often, a veterinarian will refer these cases to a board-certified veterinary ophthalmologist, who has the expertise and equipment required to treat them.

Sign/Symptom	Observations	Associated Signs	Possible Condition	Action to Take
Eyes red, watery, or with mucoid discharge	None	Possible sneezing and nasal discharge	Conjunctivitis (see Glossary), caused by an upper respiratory infection (URI—see pp. 63–64). Without respiratory signs, could be bacterial, allergic, or irritant conjunctivitis.	If not resolving, see veterinarian for eye ointment.
Third eyelid protruding (see p. 7 for description of third eyelid)	None	None. Possible diarrhea.	Idiopathic (no known cause) condition. Occasionally associated with diarrhea.	None. Usually resolves eventually.
Pupils different sizes	Possible lethargy. Pupil smaller in affected eye.	Usually none initially	Tumor (brain or eye). Trauma. Internal eye disease.	See veterinarian for examination

Call veterinarian; make appointment immediately

Life-threatening condition; go *immediately* to veterinarian or emergency clinic

Sign/Symptom	Observations	Associated Signs	Possible Condition	Action to Take
Tearing eye	May avoid light, eye may be painful	Squints	Corneal ulcer	See veterinarian for assessment, medication.
Gradual vision loss	May be reluctant to move. Bumps into things.	Possible personality changes. Possible seizures (if brain tumor).	Brain tumor. Retinal degeneration. Cataracts. Brain inflammation.	See veterinarian for examination, tests, possible referral to a veterinary ophthalmologist.
Eyes appear white or gray, opaque	Possible vision loss	None	If lens = cataracts. If cornea = edema (swelling) of cornea.	See veterinarian for diagnosis and medication for edema.
Tear streaks below eyes	Longhaired, brachycephalic cat. Chronically wet fur; eye overflows	Brown streaks on fur below eyes	Tear ducts abnormally formed or located	Antibiotics for discoloration. Ophthalmologist may be able to repair or reposition tear ducts.
Sudden vision loss	Reluctance to move, bumps into things	Lethargy	Retinal detachments (secondary to infection, hypertension)	See veterinarian for examination, tests.

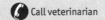

Home care; first aid   Call veterinarian   Call veterinarian; make appointment within 24 hours

Gagging

Gagging implies a throat problem and should not be confused with coughing, which comes from lower down in the airways. When a cat's throat is inflamed for any reason, mucus is produced and a gag reflex follows. A cat may gag up a small amount of foamy mucus, or may swallow the mucus once it reaches her mouth.

Sign/Symptom	Observations	Associated Signs	Possible Condition	Action to Take
Acute gagging	May swallow for no reason	None	Irritation in throat from ingested irritant (i.e., plant or drug)	See veterinarian for assessment, medication.
Acute gagging	Distressed. May paw at mouth.	Cyanosis (blue mucous membranes see Glossary)	Obstruction in throat (foreign object)	Go to emergency clinic for removal of object.
Chronic gagging	Not eating well	Bloody mucoid saliva	Foreign body (needle?). Abscess in mouth.	See veterinarian for X ray, possible surgery.
Chronic, progressive gagging	Weight loss. Anorexia. Possible lethargy.	Possible swelling in throat. Possible difficult breathing (dyspnea). Possible cyanosis (bluish mucous membranes).	Tumor or cyst in throat	See veterinarian for X ray, possible biopsy, possible surgery.
Gagging	Possible depressed appetite	Sneezing, coughing, conjunctivitis (see Glossary), possible ulcers on tongue.	Upper respiratory infection (URI—see pp. 63–64)	If eating, give supportive care. If lethargic or anorectic, see veterinarian for medication, possible fluid therapy.

 Call veterinarian; make appointment immediately   Life-threatening condition; go *immediately* to veterinarian or emergency clinic

Incoordination

A cat that is incoordinated will wobble when walking. His legs may cross and his feet may drag. This may be confined to the front or rear legs, or all four legs may be affected. Incoordination implies a neurological problem that could be affecting the brain, spinal cord, or, rarely, just the peripheral nerves (see pp. 10–11). Many brain and spinal cord disorders can only be finally diagnosed with sophisticated tests such as CAT scans and MRI's (see Glossary for definitions).

Sign/Symptom	Observations	Associated Signs	Possible Condition	Action to Take
Rear legs incoordinated	Slowly progressive	Possible back pain	Spinal cord lesion. Tumor (especially lymphoma—see Glossary). Disc disease. Vertebral instability.	See veterinarian for X rays, tests.
Rear legs incoordinated	Rapid onset	Back pain	Trauma to back. Acute disc disease. Embolus (blood clot).	Go to emergency clinic for X rays, tests.
Rear legs paralyzed or very weak	Acute onset (Note: Although this is not a neurological disease, the loss of blood supply to the rear legs will cause an inability to move.)	Panting. In pain. Crying.	Aortic embolus (blood clot), secondary to heart disease (see p. 52)	Go to emergency clinic for treatment.

Home care; first aid   Call veterinarian   Call veterinarian; make appointment within 24 hours

Sign/Symptom	Observations	Associated Signs	Possible Condition	Action to Take
All four legs incoordinated	Slow onset	Possible neck pain	Cervical (neck) spinal cord disease. Tumor (especially lymphoma—see Glossary). Instability of vertebrae. Possible fungal granuloma. Possible brain disease.	See veterinarian for X rays, CAT scan, MRI (see Glossary).
All four legs incoordinated	Rapid onset	Vomiting and/or diarrhea. Depression. Possible fever. Possible seizures.	Poisoning (drug toxicity—see pp. 50–51). Vascular insult to brain. With fever = encephalitis (see Glossary)	Go to emergency clinic. Call ASPCA National Animal Poison Control Center at 800-548-2423.
		(Note: Information on possible drug ingested is extremely helpful.)		
All four legs incoordinated	Slow onset	Personality changes. Seizures. Possible blindness. May walk in circles or fall to one side.	Brain tumor	See veterinarian for tests, CAT scan, MRI (see Glossary), and to discuss treatment options.
Staggers and falls to one side	May not eat well. Crouches. Walks along wall.	Possible head tilt	Middle- or inner-ear disease. Tumor. Infection. Feline vestibular (balance) syndrome.	See veterinarian for X rays, tests.

INCOORDINATION

Call veterinarian; make appointment immediately   Life-threatening condition; go *immediately* to veterinarian or emergency clinic

Lameness

Lameness is a condition that can have many causes. It can arise due to a simple twisted joint, similar to a sprained ankle in humans, or may have a deeper underlying cause. It can also stem from a sore, irritated paw or footpad, or a torn claw.

A cat is lame if she changes her gait to shift weight and make it less painful to use the sore leg. Because they are so nimble and well coordinated, cats can get around very well using only three legs. Therefore, a cat will usually make it easy to tell which leg is involved because she will avoid putting weight on it by holding it up.

An owner may be tempted to examine his cat's leg to try to determine the location and cause of the problem. This is not a good idea with most cats, because even good-natured cats will often bite if they are in pain. If a cat seems to be feeling well in general, it is all right to wait a day or so and see if the lameness subsides. On the other hand, if a cat is clearly ill or the lameness continues, it is best to let a veterinarian examine her.

Sign/Symptom	Observations	Associated Signs	Possible Condition	Action to Take
Lame on one leg	Lethargic. Leg painful.	Swelling of leg. Fever (see pp. 73–74 for how to take a cat's temperature). Possibly draining pus.	Abscess, almost always due to bite wound.	See veterinarian for medication, drainage of abscess.
Painful on multiple legs	Lethargic. Possible anorexia.	Possible joint swelling. Possible fever (see pp. 73–74 for how to take a cat's temperature).	Systemic disease. Arthritis. Myositis (inflamed muscle).	See veterinarian for tests, medication.

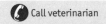 Home care; first aid   Call veterinarian   Call veterinarian; make appointment within 24 hours

Sign/Symptom	Observations	Associated Signs	Possible Condition	Action to Take
Lame on one or more legs	Outdoor cat	Swelling on lame legs. Possible scrapes on cat.	Traumatic injury (e.g., fracture, dislocation, bruise, hematoma), often secondary to being hit by car.	See veterinarian for X rays, treatment.
Progressive lameness on one leg	Possible lethargy	Usually none	Tumor. Arthritis.	See veterinarian for X rays.
Acute lameness in one leg	No fever. May or may not have known trauma.	None	Soft-tissue injury. (If rear leg, cruciate ligament rupture; sprain; strain). Orthopedic injury (dislocation; fracture).	See veterinarian for X rays, treatment.
Lame on one leg	Reluctant to move. Possible painful back or neck.	None	Pain from spinal cord lesion, caused by a tumor, trauma, pinched nerve.	See veterinarian for X rays, medication, possible surgery.

Claw Care

Cats' claws grow remarkably fast. Cats that are allowed outdoors usually wear their claws down some when they climb on rough wood surfaces. Indoor-only cats may keep their front claws reasonably short and dull if they use a rough scratching post, such as one covered with rope. But their rear claws are never worn down. If claws are allowed to become too long, they easily catch on things such as rugs, furniture, blankets, screening, etc., and may cause a cat to wrench her leg trying to get loose. Older indoor cats may stop using a scratching device altogether and can develop overgrown claws on all four legs. Owners should be aware of the potential for injury to a cat (to say nothing of the potential for damage to household furnishings, other pets, and even people) and keep a cat's claws trimmed. See pp. 29–30 for how to do this.

Call veterinarian; make appointment immediately

 Life-threatening condition; go *immediately* to veterinarian or emergency clinic

Mammary Gland Abnormalities

Cats have a total of eight mammary glands, four on each side. In young cats, males, and spayed females, these glands appear only as tiny specks. In nursing females and older female cats that have had litters of kittens, the glands may become more noticeable. As we mentioned on pp. 11 and 20–21, early spaying (before the first heat) helps prevent the later development of mammary gland tumors in female cats. Any unspayed female cat, or a spayed cat that has gone through some heat periods, should be regularly examined for masses in her breasts.

Sign/Symptom	Observations	Associated Signs	Possible Condition	Action to Take
Increased size in mammary glands	Unspayed female. May have milk in glands.	Increased size of abdomen	Pregnancy	📞 See veterinarian for confirmation and instructions.
Increase in size of one or more glands	Young pregnant cat, usually	Possible ulceration of skin of that gland	Mammary hyperplasia (enlargement)	Resolves after kittens delivered.
One or more glands hot, swollen, painful	Nursing cat	Fever (see pp. 73–74 for how to take a cat's temperature). Milk from that gland a different color.	Mastitis (infection of mammary gland)	📞 See veterinarian for antibiotic, possible lancing. ➕ Hot packs may help. ➕ That gland must not be used by kittens to nurse.
Firm masses in one or more glands	Growing in size	None	Mammary gland tumor	📞24 See veterinarian for biopsy, surgery, possible chemotherapy, possible spay.

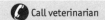

➕ Home care; first aid   📞 Call veterinarian   📞24 Call veterinarian; make appointment within 24 hours

Mouth Disorders

It is a good idea for an owner to look inside his cat's mouth to see what it normally looks like. An owner who brushes his cat's teeth on a regular basis (see p. 31) will probably detect mouth problems before they become too serious. An owner who does not perform tooth brushing should examine his cat's mouth from time to time, looking at the teeth, along the gum lines, and underneath the tongue for bleeding, redness, swelling, or other abnormalities. The most common signs associated with oral disease are foul breath, drooling, and occasionally anorexia. Bad breath can also be a sign of a systemic disorder, such as kidney disease.

Sign/Symptom	Observations	Associated Signs	Possible Condition	Action to Take
Drooling, bad breath	Depressed appetite	Possibly bloody saliva	Severe dental disease. Severe gum disease. Tumor. Abscess.	See veterinarian for treatment.
Pawing at mouth	Possible anorexia	Drooling	Foreign body (possibly a bone) caught in mouth. Severe gingival disease or loose tooth displaced.	See veterinarian for examination.
Bad breath	Lethargic. Anorectic. Weight loss.	Drinking and urinating more, eating less. Possible vomiting.	Kidney disease	See veterinarian for tests. Bring urine sample.
Small, dark permanent areas on lips, gums	Usually orange cat	None	Normal pigment change	None

Sign/Symptom	Observations	Associated Signs	Possible Condition	Action to Take
Irregular growth on gums	Older cat. Growth becoming larger.	Possible drooling	Gum tumor	See veterinarian for possible biopsy and surgery, and to discuss therapy options.
Ulcerated areas on upper lip in front of canine teeth	None	None	Eosinophilic granulomas (see Glossary), also called rodent ulcers	See veterinarian for medication.
Cannot close mouth	Mouth constantly open	Anorexia. Not drinking. Dehydration if chronic.	Loose molar tooth in back of mouth. Jaw fracture. Peripheral nerve (5th cranial nerve) disorder.	See veterinarian for assessment, possible X ray.

Feline Gum Disease

Cats have a high incidence of gum disease. Sometimes it is secondary to tartar formation. Some cats have chronic gingivitis (inflamed, bleeding gums) because of a previous infection with a respiratory virus. These cats usually have a bright red line on the gums, along the top of the teeth. This chronic inflammation may lead to tartar formation and gum recession.

Home care; first aid   Call veterinarian   Call veterinarian; make appointment within 24 hours

Mucous Membrane Color

One of the best ways to ascertain the condition of a cat is to examine his mucous membranes. The easiest, fastest way to do this is to look at the gums by simply lifting the upper lip. A cat should have pink gums that lighten if pressed and then turn normally pink again. It is a good idea for an owner to look at her pet's mouth when the animal is well, to see what the cat's normal gum color is. A second place to look for mucous membrane color is the eye. The white part (sclera) should be white, and the inside of the lower lid (conjunctiva) pink. Additionally, many cats have pink noses that also change color along with the mucous membranes.

When a cat is dehydrated her skin will lose its elasticity and will not bounce back immediately when grasped, but will tent momentarily. Dehydration occurs when there is a decreased intake of water for whatever reason, or increased water loss due to illness or high fever.

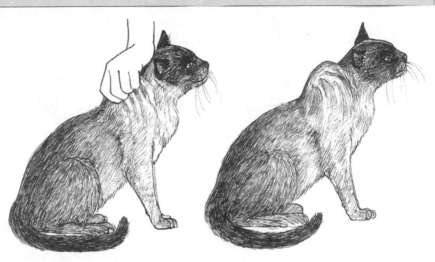

Sign/Symptom	Observations	Associated Signs	Possible Condition	Action to Take
Pale pink mucous membranes	Possible lethargy. Possible anorexia.	Possible diarrhea. Possible vomiting.	Dehydration	See veterinarian for tests, fluids.
Bright-red mucous membranes	Feels warm. Temperature over 103 degrees (see pp. 73–74 for how to take a cat's temperature).	Anorexia. Lethargy.	Fever (infection; FeLV [see pp. 61–62]; FIV [see p. 61]; tumor)	See veterinarian for tests, medication.

 Call veterinarian; make appointment immediately

Life-threatening condition; go *immediately* to veterinarian or emergency clinic

Sign/Symptom	Observations	Associated Signs	Possible Condition	Action to Take
Purple/blue mucous membranes	Not moving. Nose and tongue also purple.	Labored breathing. Possible cough. Possible fever.	Heart failure (see p. 52). Lung problem (tumor, trauma, asthma, pneumonia). Fluid in chest (see "Respiratory Difficulties"). Acetaminophen ingestion.	Go to emergency clinic for X rays, tests, oxygen.
Yellow mucous membranes	Usually lethargic, anorectic. Inside of ear pinna may look yellow. Whites of eyes yellow.	Possible vomiting	Liver disease (tumor, inflammation, fatty infiltration, FIP [see p. 61], secondary to cardiac disease, peritonitis, pancreatic disease). Hemolytic anemia (see Glossary) due to drugs, immune-mediated disease, hemobartonella (see Glossary).	See veterinarian for tests, X rays, possible ultrasound, possible biopsy.
Pale to white mucous membranes. Pale nose.	Lethargic. Depressed. Acute or gradual onset.	Usually none. Rarely— dark stools from gastrointestinal bleeding, or chronic bloody urine. If bleeding is severe, difficulty breathing.	Anemia (FeLV [see pp. 61–62]; FIV [see p. 61]; tumor; blood loss; rat poison [see p. 50]; chronic kidney failure; immune-mediated disease; drug ingestion [see p. 50]).	Go to emergency clinic for tests, transfusion
Pale mucous membranes	Depressed. Labored breathing. Acute onset.	None	Shock (see p. 55) due to: cardiac disease (see p. 52), trauma, blood loss, severe bacterial infection.	Go to emergency clinic for fluids, medication. Treat underlying disease.

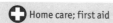 Home care; first aid 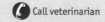 Call veterinarian 24 Call veterinarian; make appointment within 24 hours

Nasal Disorders,
Including Changes in the Nares

There are a number of nasal disorders that are characterized by a discharge, either watery, bloody, mucoid, or purulent (containing pus). There are others that change the appearance of the nose. The inner nasal passages are very difficult to examine. In order to obtain samples for diagnosis, a cat may need to be anesthetized so that fluid can be flushed up her nose, and the retrieved fluid evaluated. A nasoscope may also be used to examine the inner portions of the nose. Other valuable diagnostic tools are a CAT scan (see Glossary) or MRI (also see Glossary).

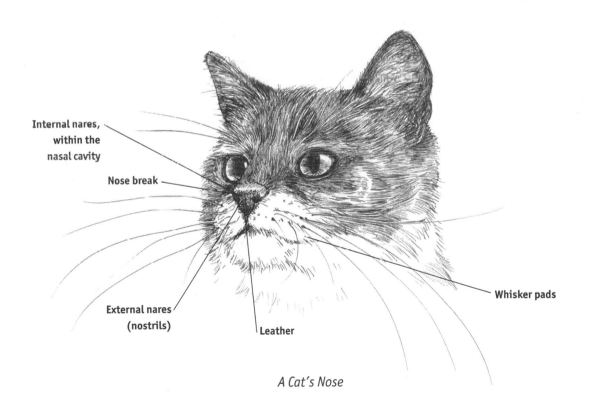

Internal nares, within the nasal cavity

Nose break

External nares (nostrils)

Leather

Whisker pads

A Cat's Nose

 Call veterinarian; make appointment immediately

Life-threatening condition; go *immediately* to veterinarian or emergency clinic

Sign/Symptom	Observations	Associated Signs	Possible Condition	Action to Take
Bilateral mucoid nasal discharge	Possible lethargy. Possible anorexia.	Conjunctivitis (see Glossary). Sneezing. Possible cough. Possible fever (see pp. 73–74 for how to take a cat's temperature).	Upper respiratory virus	✚ If eating and feeling well, wait a few days. 🕓 If anorectic or feeling poorly, see veterinarian for medication, possible X ray.
Bilateral mucoid or purulent nasal discharge	Anorexia. Possible lethargy.	Labored breathing. Sneezing. Fever (see pp. 73–74).	Pneumonia (bacterial, fungal, viral)	⊕ Go to emergency clinic for assessment, medication.
Chronic bilateral mucoid, purulent, or bloody nasal discharge	Nasal discharge sneezed (found) around the house.	Sneezing	Sinusitis (bacterial, fungal)	📞 See veterinarian for tests, medication.
Bilateral or unilateral bloody, mucoid, or purulent discharge	Progressively worsening. May see change in contour of nose.	None	Nasal tumor. Foreign body in nose. Bone infection.	📞 See veterinarian for X ray, MRI, CAT scan (see Glossary), possible nasoscope.
Bilateral or unilateral watery nasal discharge	None	May have upper respiratory infection (URI—see pp. 63–64), or conjunctivitis (see Glossary)	Excessive tears discharging from nose (see Box, below)	📞 See veterinarian to treat underlying disease.
Scabby lesions on nares	Usually white or light-colored cats. Progressively becoming worse.	May have similar lesions on eyelids and/or ears	Tumor (squamous cell carcinoma—see Glossary)	📞 See veterinarian to discuss options.

✚ Home care; first aid   📞 Call veterinarian   🕓 Call veterinarian; make appointment within 24 hours

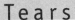

Tears

Tears are carried from the eyes to the nose via small ducts. The normal amount of tears is not noticeable but contributes to keeping the nasal membranes moist. Excessive tearing causes dripping from the nose.

Sinusitis in Cats

Sinusitis in cats may occur secondarily to an upper respiratory infection (URI—see pp. 63–64). It may be extremely difficult to treat and many cats live their entire lives with it controlled only to a small degree. One uncommon form of sinusitis is caused by a fungus (cryptococcosis—see p. 65), which can infect humans. This should be eliminated as a possible diagnosis in any cat with a chronic nasal discharge.

Call veterinarian; make appointment immediately

Life-threatening condition; go *immediately* to veterinarian or emergency clinic

Rectal Problems

Cats rarely have serious rectal problems. However, they do occasionally have anal sac disease and hernias.

Sign/Symptom	Observations	Associated Signs	Possible Condition	Action to Take
Red/purple area to side of rectum	May be reluctant to move bowels	Possible fever (see pp. 73–74 for how to take a cat's temperature)	Anal sac abscess	See veterinarian to drain, give antibiotics.
Scoots along floor/ ground on rectum, or licks at rectum.	None	None	Nonspecific rectal irritation. Often due to anal sac impaction/ infection or diarrhea, causing rectal irritation. Longhaired cats with diarrhea may have soft stool caught in the hair by the rectum, which can cause irritation.	See veterinarian to examine and treat anal sacs.
Blood from rectum	May move bowels frequently	Mucoid stool	Colitis due to: parasites, foreign material, dietary allergy, infection, tumor	See veterinarian. Bring stool sample.
Blood on stool	Stool fairly normal	None	Rectal or colonic polyp or tumor. Rectal crack.	See veterinarian for rectal examination, tests.
Bulge to side of rectum	Strains to move bowels	None	Perineal hernia (near or around the anus). Anal sac abscess.	See veterinarian for treatment options.

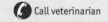 Home care; first aid   Call veterinarian   Call veterinarian; make appointment within 24 hours

Respiratory Difficulties

Respiratory difficulties include common problems that prevent a cat from getting sufficient oxygen when she breathes. Normally a cat with this difficulty will be lethargic and may cough. The most common serious sign of respiratory difficulty is what is called abdominal breathing. The cat's abdominal muscles play a limited role in normal respiration. If more negative pressure is needed by a cat in order to inhale, her abdominal muscles will be called into play, and an owner will clearly see the animal's stomach expand whenever she inhales. *A cat with respiratory difficulties should not be subjected to a hot environment.*

Reverse Sneezing

Although common in dogs, cats only occasionally have bouts of reverse sneezing. Because this is not a human action, owners have difficulty describing what happens. It seems to be an asthmatic attack, or the inability of a cat to catch her breath. It sounds as if the cat is repeatedly snorting. In reality, it is a series of spasmodic, rapid inhalations through the nose. Cats usually go from acting perfectly normal to having an episode of reverse sneezing that lasts for about thirty seconds.

Reverse sneezing is caused by an irritation in the pharynx. Anything that causes irritation in the windpipe will trigger an attack. Normally, it is associated with allergies or sore throats and is more common in brachycephalic breeds. Often, feeding a cat soft foods will alleviate the problem. If it becomes severe, the veterinarian may prescribe anti-inflammatory drugs and antibiotics.

Call veterinarian; make appointment immediately

Life-threatening condition; go *immediately* to veterinarian or emergency clinic

Sign/Symptom	Observations	Associated Signs	Possible Condition	Action to Take
Labored breathing	Lethargic, depressed appetite	Mucoid nasal discharge. Fever. Possible conjunctivitis (see Glossary). Possible sneezing. Possible ulcers on tongue. Cough.	Respiratory virus. Pneumonia.	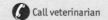 See veterinarian for assessment, medication, possible X ray.
Labored breathing	Lethargic. Depressed appetite. Possible weight loss and cough.	Possible fever. Cyanotic tongue (see Glossary).	Fluid in chest due to: cardiac problems (see p. 52); cancer (especially FeLV-related [see pp. 61–62]); chylothorax; pyrothorax (pus in chest); FIP (see p. 61). Tumor. Fungal infection. Pneumonia. Lung-worms. Heartworm.	Go to emergency clinic for tests, X ray.

Coughing

When a cat coughs it is a rather nonspecific sign, and could be due to any of the above-mentioned diseases or disorders. The most common reasons a cat coughs are asthma, upper respiratory infections (URI's, see pp. 63–64), and lung worm infection. Cats with hair balls may appear to cough, but this is actually gagging and retching.

Home care; first aid   Call veterinarian   Call veterinarian; make appointment within 24 hours

Sign/Symptom	Observations	Associated Signs	Possible Condition	Action to Take
Mild to severe labored breathing	May come and go. Lethargic when having difficulty.	Cough, possible cyanosis (blue mucous membranes)	Feline asthma	to Depending on severity, see veterinarian, or go to emergency clinic for X ray and to discuss treatment and prevention options.
Severe labored breathing	Very distressed. Will not move.	Cyanotic tongue. Possible foamy nasal discharge, cough.	Acute cardiac failure; severe asthma	Go to emergency clinic for medication, oxygen, tests.
Labored breathing	Depressed. Lethargic. Anorexic.	Pale mucous membranes	Anemia due to: FeLV (see pp. 62–63); tumor; kidney disease; trauma; rat poison; drugs (see pp. 50–51)	Go to emergency clinic for tests, possible transfusion.

Panting

Panting is rapid, shallow, open-mouthed breathing. Cats that pant almost always are either nervous or in severe pain. It should not be difficult to determine which is the case. Cats may also pant when overheated but, compared with dogs, this is relatively rare.

Call veterinarian; make appointment immediately

 Life-threatening condition; go *immediately* to veterinarian or emergency clinic

Sign/Symptom	Observations	Associated Signs	Possible Condition	Action to Take
Labored breathing	History of trauma	Signs of trauma, cuts, abrasions. Possible cough.	Bleeding into lungs. Collapsed lung. Pneumothorax (air in chest). Diaphragmatic hernia (rip in diaphragm allowing abdominal organs to move into chest).	Go to emergency clinic for X rays, medication, possible surgery.
Labored breathing	Burn on mouth or tongue possible. Electric cord damaged.	Collapse	Pulmonary edema secondary to electrocution	Go to emergency clinic for treatments, oxygen.

Home care; first aid   Call veterinarian   Call veterinarian; make appointment within 24 hours

Skin Disorders

This is an extremely broad category. The areas covered include: changes in the skin, including lumps and bumps; changes that cause pruritis (itching) or rashes; and conditions that cause hair loss or color change.

The underlying causes of skin problems can be very difficult to diagnose. There are veterinarians who specialize in dermatology who may be consulted in very difficult or persistent cases.

Sign/Symptom	Observations	Associated Signs	Possible Condition	Action to Take
Solitary mass, increasing in size	None	None	Tumor or cyst	See veterinarian for biopsy, possible surgery.
	(Note: A higher percentage of cutaneous [skin] masses are malignant in the cat as opposed to the dog. Any mass that is growing should be viewed as a potential problem not to be ignored.)			
Ulcerated growths on ears, nose	Usually white cats	May scratch at them, causing bleeding	Tumor (usually squamous cell carcinoma—see Glossary)	See veterinarian for biopsy, surgery, other options.
Itchy face, ears	Scratches at head, causing ulceration and redness, rubbing face on furniture, causing irritation	None	Allergic reaction (usually to food). Mange. Ear mites.	See veterinarian for examination, medication.
Small scabs along back and head	Hair sparse along back	Some itching	Miliary dermatitis (allergic reaction, usually to fleas or food—see Box, p. 131). Occasionally there is a bacterial component.	See veterinarian for medication.

Call veterinarian; make appointment immediately   Life-threatening condition; go *immediately* to veterinarian or emergency clinic

Sign/Symptom	Observations	Associated Signs	Possible Condition	Action to Take
Red, ulcerated areas, often inside thighs	May see cat licking at them	None	Eosinophilic plaques (see Glossary)	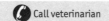 See veterinarian for medication.
Bloody discharge from side of rectum	May be painful to move bowels	Possible fever (see pp. 73–74 for how to take a cat's temperature)	Anal sac abscess (see also "Rectal Problems")	See veterinarian to drain, give antibiotics.
Swelling anywhere (legs, head, tail area). Acute onset.	May be lethargic. Area painful and hot.	May be draining pus. Fever.	Abscess, usually due to bite wound	See veterinarian to drain, give antibiotics.
Abdominal hair loss	Potbelly. Eating and drinking more.	Possible increased thirst and urination if secondary diabetes mellitus develops	Cushing's syndrome (see Glossary)	See veterinarian for tests. Discuss treatment.
Progressive hair loss on groin and rear legs	May see cat licking hair out	None	Allergic reaction or behavioral (stress related)	See veterinarian for medication.
Mats and dandruff along back	Cat may be obese	None	Improper grooming by cat (obese, sick, or lazy)	Comb cat regularly.
Skin yellow	Lethargic. Anorectic.	Possible vomiting	Liver disease (fatty liver, FIP [see pp. 60–61], inflammatory disease, tumor, infection, or hemolytic anemia). Peritonitis. Pancreatic disease.	See veterinarian for tests.
Single or multiple round, hairless areas anywhere on body; possibly flaky	Usually not pruritic (itchy)	People in home (especially children) may have skin lesions	Ringworm (fungal dermatitis)	See veterinarian for treatment, possibly shaving cat.

(Note: Cats can carry ringworm without having visible lesions themselves. Sometimes these cats will develop lesions with stress or illness.)

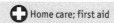 Home care; first aid   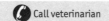 Call veterinarian   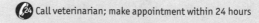 Call veterinarian; make appointment within 24 hours

Flea Infestations and Miliary Dermatitis

Miliary dermatitis manifests itself as small, red, crusty skin lesions, and is the most annoying manifestation of a flea infestation to a cat. It may be the only indication that an owner sees of a flea infestation. Often, cats do not seem to be particularly bothered by fleas, and may not scratch much. Although this is fine for the cat it gives little warning to owners of the impending flea infestation of the house or other pets. It is a good idea to check cats for fleas periodically. The best way to do this is to run a flea comb through the hair on the cat's spine near the tail and look for fleas or flea dirt, which is the black, hard fecal material of the flea.

Cats and Grooming

The most difficult places for a cat to reach to groom are the middle of her back and her rump, near the tail. Normal grooming with a cat's rough tongue will remove dead hair and skin. Some cats are not fastidious and have no interest in grooming themselves. They must be regularly groomed by their owners. Of course, very fat cats just cannot reach many areas and need help to stay well groomed. If a cat has always been a good, thorough groomer and suddenly stops grooming herself, it may be a sign of a medical problem.

 Call veterinarian; make appointment immediately   Life-threatening condition; go *immediately* to veterinarian or emergency clinic

Straining to Move Bowels

When a cat is straining to move his bowels, either he is constipated or he has colitis (large bowel diarrhea). An owner should determine if the cat is producing frequent soft, mucoid, sometimes bloody stool (colitis), or pieces of very hard stool (constipation).

Owners may very easily confuse straining to move bowels with straining to urinate. When a male cat is straining, it is important to be sure he is producing urine. If an owner cannot be sure, and the cat appears to be in discomfort, it is possible he has a urinary obstruction and *he should be examined by a veterinarian immediately*. See also "Urination, Abnormal."

Sign/Symptom	Observations	Associated Signs	Possible Condition	Action to Take
Straining to move bowels	In and out of litter box, squats, strains	Small amounts of mucoid stool, sometimes with blood	Colitis due to: food allergy, parasites, dietary indiscretion (especially plants), tumors.	✚ See "Home Treatment for Routine Diarrhea or Vomiting," p. 106. 📞 If persists, see veterinarian. Bring fecal sample for tests.
Straining to move bowels	Any stool passed is very hard	Possible vomiting, dehydration	Constipation, usually not a primary problem, secondary to dehydration from another illness	📞24 See veterinarian for examination, tests, fluids, medication, possible enema.
Straining to move bowels	May have swelling to side of rectum. Stool passed is fairly normal.	May have fever (see pp. 73–74 for how to take a cat's temperature)	Perianal hernia. If fever = anal sac abscess.	📞24 See veterinarian for rectal exam. If abscess = possible antibiotics and drainage. If hernia = usually surgery.

✚ Home care; first aid   📞 Call veterinarian   📞24 Call veterinarian; make appointment within 24 hours

Sign/Symptom	Observations	Associated Signs	Possible Condition	Action to Take
Acute straining to move bowels	No bowel movement seen in 1–2 days	Anorexia. Dehydration. Vomiting. Increased thirst and urination.	Constipation usually not a primary problem—often associated with dehydration from another illness.	See veterinarian for tests, treatment, fluids.
Chronic straining to move bowels	No stool, or scant stool is passed	If chronic, may lead to anorexia, vomiting, dehydration	Rectal stricture. Obstipation (megacolon).	See veterinarian for enemas, deobstipation, stool softeners, possible surgery.

Call veterinarian; make appointment immediately   Life-threatening condition; go *immediately* to veterinarian or emergency clinic

Thirst, Changes in

When a cat drinks an excessive amount of water, it must be excreted from her body in urine. Therefore, increased thirst and urination go hand in hand. An owner may notice that the litter requires more frequent changing. Conversely, if a cat is producing too much urine for a variety of medical reasons, she must drink more than she normally does or she will become dehydrated. This condition is known as polyuria (excessive urination)/polydipsia (excessive thirst), or PU/PD. Of course, if a cat is an indoor-outdoor or strictly outdoor pet and does not use a litter pan, it can be difficult, if not impossible, for an owner to notice increased urination.

Sign/Symptom	Observations	Associated Signs	Possible Condition	Action to Take
PU/PD	Increased appetite	Weight loss	Diabetes mellitus. Hyperthyroidism (see Glossary)	See veterinarian for tests, treatment (normally, insulin injections for diabetes; medication, surgery, or radiotherapy for hyperthyroidism).
PU/PD	Hair loss. Increased size of abdomen.	Increased appetite.	Diabetes mellitus secondary to Cushing's syndrome (see Glossary).	See veterinarian for tests, treatment.
PU/PD	None	None	May be psychogenic (originating in the mind). Diabetes insipidus.	See veterinarian for tests, possible treatment. If psychogenic = behavior modification.

Home care; first aid   Call veterinarian   Call veterinarian; make appointment within 24 hours

Sign/Symptom	Observations	Associated Signs	Possible Condition	Action to Take
PU/PD	Appetite poor. Weight loss.	Nausea/vomiting. Possible mouth odor.	Kidney disease (infection, degeneration, tumor), hypocalcemia	(24) See veterinarian for tests, fluids, medication, possible prescription diet.
PU/PD	Unspayed female. Cat very sick, lethargic, anorexic.	Fever (see pp. 73–74 for how to take a cat's temperature). Possible distended abdomen. Possible vaginal discharge.	Pyometra (see p. 53; see also Box, p. 97)	(i) See veterinarian for X rays, tests, surgery.

(i) Call veterinarian; make appointment immediately   (+) Life-threatening condition; go *immediately* to veterinarian or emergency clinic

Urination, Abnormal

When a cat strains to urinate or produces abnormal urine there are always underlying medical causes. In male cats, it is potentially an extremely serious problem because, if they have a bladder inflammation, they may produce crystals that obstruct the urethra (tube that carries urine out of the body from the bladder). These cats strain and produce no urine. See also "Urinary Emergencies," p. 54. As we said in "Thirst, Changes in," above, it may be difficult for owners of cats that go outdoors and do not use a litter box to observe any changes in urination. They will have to rely on other signs of trouble.

Sign/Symptom	Observations	Associated Signs	Possible Condition	Action to Take
Straining to urinate. Produces a small amount of urine.	In and out of litter box. Eating well and acting normal.	Urine may be bloody	Bladder infection/inflammation	See veterinarian for examination, medication, possible diet change. Bring urine sample if possible.
Straining to urinate	Male cat. No urine produced. Anorectic. May cry if picked up.	Possible vomiting	Urinary obstruction (stones/crystals; rarely, trauma or tumor)	Go to emergency clinic for bladder catheterization, medication, fluids, possible X rays, possible diet change.
Bloody urine	History of trauma	None	Trauma to bladder or ruptured bladder	See veterinarian for X rays, tests, surgery if ruptured.
Leaking urine when lying down	Generally progressive	Possibly weak rear legs	Incontinence (spinal cord disease; FeLV-related [see pp. 61–62]); endocrine disorder	See veterinarian for X rays, tests.

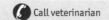

Home care; first aid   Call veterinarian   Call veterinarian; make appointment within 24 hours

Sign/Symptom	Observations	Associated Signs	Possible Condition	Action to Take
Spraying urine (see "Territorial Behavior," pp. 35–36; see also "Elimination Behavior," p. 39)	Usually, but not always, male cat, either neutered or intact	Urine found on vertical surfaces	Territorial marking	See veterinarian or behaviorist to discuss behavior modification, medication, or deterrents.
Urination in inappropriate locations	Normal amounts of urine, often in the same places	Urine found on vertical surfaces	Behavioral (stress-related; genetic; litter or litter box location avoidance—see "Housebreaking Problems," pp. 41–42)	See veterinarian or behaviorist to discuss behavior modification, medication, deterrents.
Dark-yellow urine	Weight loss. Lethargy. Anorexia.	Possible vomiting, jaundice (see Glossary)	Liver disease (fatty liver; FIP [see pp. 60–61]; tumor—infectious or inflammatory); peritonitis; pancreatic disease	See veterinarian for tests.

U

R
I
N
A
T
I
O
N
,

A
B
N
O
R
M
A
L

Call veterinarian; make appointment immediately

Life-threatening condition; go *immediately* to veterinarian or emergency clinic

Vomiting

Vomiting is the big brother of nausea. Often, before vomiting occurs, an owner will notice a cat's lack of interest in most food, or an interest only in some food the animal really likes. The cat may also drool. These are signs of nausea. Sometimes, the condition resolves itself before the cat actually vomits. But if the stomach or intestines are severely irritated, the cat will eventually vomit. Often, a cat that vomits will also develop diarrhea because if her stomach is irritated from something ingested, the irritating substance will pass through the digestive tract into her intestines.

Cats often yowl before or after vomiting. This is assumed to be a pain response.

Most cases of vomiting are not emergencies, with the exceptions of: urinary tract obstructions in male cats (see "Urination, Abnormal"); the ingestion of linear objects (string, thread, ribbon, tinsel, etc.); and peritonitis (inflammation of membranes lining the abdominal cavity). However, severe vomiting and diarrhea from any cause will eventually lead to dehydration and electrolyte imbalances that can be life-threatening. *If any vomiting cat becomes noticeably lethargic, it is an emergency.* See p. 106, "Home Treatment of Routine Diarrhea or Vomiting."

Sign/Symptom	Observations	Associated Signs	Possible Condition	Action to Take
Acute to occasional vomiting	Usually kittens. Long, spaghettilike worms in vomitus.	Possibly potbellied. Possible diarrhea.	Roundworms	See veterinarian for confirmation, medication. Take fecal sample.
Acute to sporadic vomiting	Eating houseplants, fabric. Hunting cats eating prey.	Drooling. Possible lethargy. Normal stools or diarrhea.	Foreign body causing irritation	Home care for vomiting (see Box, p. 106). If persists, see veterinarian for medication, X rays.

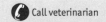

V

O
M
I
T
I
N
G

Sign/Symptom	Observations	Associated Signs	Possible Condition	Action to Take
Frequent, acute vomiting	History, or reasonable possibility, of ingestion of: plastic, fabric, or linear foreign body (thread, string, ribbon, etc.). Depressed.	No stool, or diarrhea	Intestinal obstruction or linear foreign material causing severe intestinal damage	Go to emergency clinic for tests, X rays, surgery.
Acute vomiting. Rapid onset.	History of possible drug ingestion, plant ingestion	Possible diarrhea. Possible neurological signs. Possible anemia.	Intoxication	Go to emergency clinic for fluids, specific treatment. Call ASPCA National Animal Poison Control Center, 800-548-2423.
Chronic, progressive vomiting	Muscle wasting. Weight loss. Possible depression. Possible abdominal distension.	Possible diarrhea. Possible jaundice (see Glossary).	Abdominal cancer (liver, spleen, stomach, intestines, kidneys). Organ failure (liver, kidneys).	See veterinarian for tests, X rays, possible ultrasound.
Vomiting with blood	Blood mixed with vomitus, often flecks or clots	Possible dark stools. Possible anemia.	Gastric ulcer. Gastric tumor. Gastric foreign body. Rat poison or drug ingestion (see pp. 50–51).	See veterinarian for tests, possible endoscopy, transfusion.
Chronic, episodic vomiting	Slow, or no, weight loss	Possible diarrhea	Older cat—inflammatory bowel disease (IBD—see Glossary). Dietary allergy or indiscretion.	See veterinarian for examination, tests.
Chronic, intermittent vomiting	Occurs 1–3 times per week	Normal appetite. *No weight loss.*	May be normal in some cats. Possible dietary sensitivity.	Observe for other signs. Change diet.

 Call veterinarian; make appointment immediately   Life-threatening condition; go *immediately* to veterinarian or emergency clinic

Sign/Symptom	Observations	Associated Signs	Possible Condition	Action to Take
Episodic vomiting	Old cat. Ravenous appetite. Weight loss. Possibly nervous.	Possible diarrhea	Hyperthyroidism (see Glossary)	🕿 See veterinarian for examination, blood tests, treatment options.
Vomiting, acute	Male cat. Straining to urinate, in and out of litter box. Depressed. Anorectic.	May show pain if picked up	Urinary tract obstruction	✚ Go to emergency clinic to relieve obstruction, give medication, fluids.
Vomits occasionally	Longhaired cats especially. May vomit cigar-shaped wads of hair.	May yowl or caterwaul before vomiting	Hair balls	✚ Groom cat regularly. ✚ Use veterinarian-approved hair ball medication, designed to lubricate swallowed hair and move it into the bowels.
Vomiting	Lethargy	Diarrhea. Fever (see pp. 73–74 for how to take a cat's temperature).	Infection, bacterial or viral. Inflammatory bowel disease (IBD). See Glossary.	🕿 See veterinarian for tests, medication.

✚ Home care; first aid 🕿 Call veterinarian 🕿24 Call veterinarian; make appointment within 24 hours

Causes of Vomiting in Cats

When a cat has an acute vomiting or diarrhea attack and seems to be fine otherwise, try to think of what she may have ingested. If she is an indoor cat, she may have eaten houseplants, or she may have changed diets. Sometimes, she may have eaten some human medication that was left out inadvertently (some cats will not eat anything of this sort; others, of a curious nature, may). A swallowed linear object (thread, etc.) can be life-threatening and will cause a cat to vomit. Another cause for upset may be an allergic reaction to some bit of food not normally eaten. Cats that go outdoors clearly have the potential to eat anything (birds may give them salmonella, for instance). If a cat that goes outdoors suddenly develops vomiting or diarrhea, it is best to keep her in for several days, for several reasons. First, she can be more easily observed and medicated. Second, an owner can see what her stools are like. Third, she will be kept from getting into more digestive difficulty. See p. 106, "Home Treatment of Routine Diarrhea or Vomiting."

Call veterinarian; make appointment immediately

Life-threatening condition; go *immediately* to veterinarian or emergency clinic

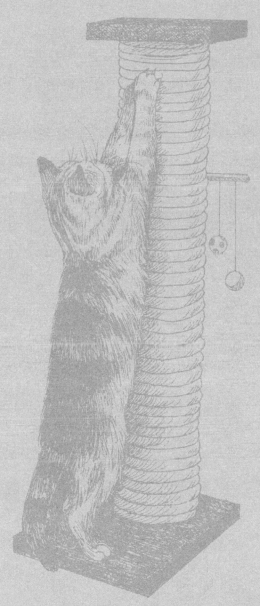

Appendixes

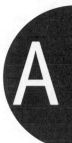

SOME COMMON HOUSEHOLD PRODUCTS THAT ARE POISONOUS

If a cat is known to have ingested any of these substances, take *immediately* to veterinarian or emergency clinic.

ASPCA National Animal Poison Control Center: 800-548-2423

Substance	Symptoms	Treatment
Acetaminophen	Blue mucous membranes, dyspnea, swollen face	Oxygen, specific antidote
Ammonium disinfectants (fabric softener)	Vomiting, diarrhea, neurological depression, seizures	Dilute of milk/water (1:1).* Activated charcoal. Saline cathartics. Supportive care for seizures, ulcers.
Antidepressant drugs	Vomiting, hyperexcitability, lack of balance, tremors, seizures, irregular heartbeat	Sedatives to counteract drug. Cardiac therapy.
Antiflea and tick pesticides (collars, sprays, powders)	Vomiting, diarrhea, lack of balance	Fluid and drug therapy
Antifreeze	Mental confusion, vomiting, collapse, kidney failure, death	*Immediate veterinary treatment essential.* Intravenous saline and bicarbonates. Activated charcoal. Specific antidotes.
Aspirin and ibuprofen	Nausea, vomiting, stomach pain, possible lethargy	Intravenous fluids. Sodium bicarbonate. Other drugs.
Bleaches	Salivation, vomiting due to ulceration	Dilute of milk/water (1:1).* Supportive care, fluids.

*May be given at home before *immediate* transportation to veterinarian or emergency clinic. Do not waste time. To induce vomiting, give 1–2 teaspoons of hydrogen peroxide (1:1 with water) or 1–2 teaspoons of syrup of ipecac.

Substance	Symptoms	Treatment
Chocolate, caffeine	Vomiting, diarrhea, hyperactivity, possible seizures	Emetics to induce vomiting.* Diazepam.
Lead (paint, toys, shot, improperly glazed bowls)	Vomiting, abdominal distress, constipation or diarrhea, muscle spasms, hysteria, blindness	Blood test. Cathartics or surgery to remove lead. Corticosteroids. Systemic or oral drug therapy.
Onions, garlic	Anemia	Blood transfusion and fluids
Petroleum distillates (gasoline, fuels, solvents, paints)	Aspiration pneumonia if inhaled; burns if skin exposure	Oxygen. Rest. If ingested: activated charcoal, gastric lavage. For burns, wash with detergent or degreaser.* Supportive care.
Rodenticides		
Anticoagulant rat poison	Anemia; nosebleeds; gastrointestinal or urinary bleeding; bruising; difficulty breathing	Vitamin K injections. Blood transfusions. 2–4 weeks of therapy.
Cholecalciferol rat poison	Depression, vomiting, weakness	Induce vomiting.* Activated charcoal. Diuretics, fluids, other drugs.
Strychnine—vole and gopher poison	Nervousness, stiffness, seizures	Activated charcoal. Sedation; gastric lavage. Diazepam or phenobarbital by IV. Fluid therapy.
Zinc phosphide	Severe gastritis, abdominal distension, vomiting, hypoglycemic shock, death	Emetics.* Absorbents. Rapid evacuation of stomach contents. Fluid therapy. Medications to reduce stomach acid.

*May be given at home before *immediate* transportation to veterinarian or emergency clinic. Do not waste time. To induce vomiting, give 1–2 teaspoons of hydrogen peroxide (1:1 with water) or 1–2 teaspoons of syrup of ipecac.

SOME CONGENITAL DEFECTS AND DISORDERS

(Note: This is *not* an exhaustive list. Most of these defects and disorders are extremely rare, and are only listed as possibilities.)

Breed/Color	Defects and/or Disorders
Abyssinian	*Amyloidosis.* The infiltration of the kidneys and liver with a starchy substance affecting kidney function and leading to kidney failure.
	Myasthenia gravis. A disease that causes muscle weakness, including an inability to blink both eyes, breathing difficulty, and regurgitation.
	*Retinal degeneration.** Degeneration of the retina at the back of the eye, leading to blindness.
Balinese	*Lysosomal storage diseases.* Brain disorders caused by an inheritable deficiency of key enzymes.
Birman	*Cataracts,** present at birth, may not be visible until 6–8 weeks of age. Juvenile cataracts may develop up to 6 years of age and heredity is usual cause. In kittens, both types of cataracts may spontaneously disappear.
	Hypotrichosis. A defect of the hair follicles leading to complete hair loss at 6 months of age.
British Shorthair	*Factor IX deficiency (hemophilia B).* A sex-linked (females) bleeding disorder, characterized by failure of normal blood clotting.
Burmese	*Endocardial fibroelastosis.* An overgrowth of elastic and fibrous fibers in the inner lining of the left atrium and ventricle of the heart. Leads to heart failure early in life.

Adapted, in part, from: *Textbook of Veterinary Internal Medicine,* Steven J. Ettinger, D.V.M., and Edward C. Feldman, D.V.M., editors. W. B. Saunders Co., Philadelphia. Appendix 2, "Congenital Defects of Cats," Johnny D. Hoskins, D.V.M.

*Prospective owners should screen parents and previous litters.

Breed/Color	Defects and/or Disorders
Canadian Hairless	*Alopecia universalis*. Lack of hair coverage.
Cornish Rex—see Rexes	
Devon Rex—see Rexes	
Domestic Shorthair	*Agenesis of the eyelid*. An absence of portions of the edge of the eyelid.
	Cataracts, * present at birth, may not be visible until 6–8 weeks of age. Juvenile cataracts may develop up to 6 years of age and heredity is usual cause. In kittens, both types of cataracts may spontaneously disappear.
	Corneal dystrophy. Corneal dullness, usually in both eyes.
	Cutaneous asthenia (Ehlers-Danlos syndrome). An abnormality of the connective tissues of the skin, resulting in loose, sagging skin that tears easily.
	Factor IX deficiency (hemophilia B). A sex-linked (females) bleeding disorder characterized by failure of normal blood clotting.
	Lysosomal storage diseases. Brain disorders caused by an inheritable deficiency of key enzymes.
	Mucopolysaccharidosis. An inherited enzyme deficiency causing lesions in the bones, brain, and eyes.
	Porphyria. An accumulation of blood pigments caused by an enzyme defect, resulting in tooth discoloration and brownish urine, which turns red under fluorescent light.
	X-linked muscular dystrophy. Causes a stiff gait ("bunny hop"). Appears at 6–9 weeks of age.
European Shorthair	*X-linked muscular dystrophy*—see Domestic Shorthair, above.
Himalayan	*Cataracts,* * present at birth, may not be visible until 6–8 weeks of age. Juvenile cataracts may develop up to 6 years of age and heredity is usual cause. In kittens, both types of cataracts may spontaneously disappear.
	Cutaneous asthenia (Ehlers-Danlos syndrome). An abnormality of the connective tissues of the skin, resulting in loose, sagging skin that tears easily.

*Prospective owners should screen parents and previous litters.

Breed/Color	Defects and/or Disorders
	von Willebrand's disease. * An inherited bleeding disorder, affecting Factor VIII and platelet function.
Korat	*Lysosomal storage diseases.* Brain disorders caused by an inheritable deficiency of key enzymes.
Maltese	*Spina bifida.* A defective fusion of spinal vertebrae, causing paralysis.
Manx	*Anury.* An absence of one to all tail vertebrae and a short, or absent, tail.
Mexican Hairless	*Hypotrichosis.* A defect of the hair follicles leading to complete hair loss at 6 months of age.
Persian	*Agenesis of the eyelid.* An absence of portions of the edge of the eyelid.
	Cataracts, * present at birth, may not be visible until 6–8 weeks of age. Juvenile cataracts may develop up to 6 years of age and heredity is usual cause. In kittens, both types of cataracts may spontaneously disappear.
	Chediak-Higashi syndrome. An immune-mediated disorder, causing susceptibility to infections, eye lesions, and abnormal bleeding.
	Entropion. Inward-turning eyelid(s), usually lower.
	Lysosomal storage diseases. Brain disorders caused by an inheritable deficiency of key enzymes.
	Patent ductus arteriosus. A condition in which a fetal blood vessel does not close at birth, causing a heart murmur and leading to heart failure.
	Polycystic kidneys. A number of fluid-filled cysts on the kidneys that may result in kidney failure.
	Retinal degeneration. * Degeneration of the retina at the back of the eye, leading to blindness.
Rexes, Cornish and Devon	*Hypotrichosis.* A defect of the hair follicles leading to complete hair loss at 6 months of age.
Siamese	*Cleft palate/cleft lip syndrome.* Midline closing defect affecting the lips and hard palate of the mouth.

*Prospective owners should screen parents and previous litters.

Breed/Color	Defects and/or Disorders
Siamese (cont'd)	*Convergent strabismus.** Crossed eyes.
	Endocardial fibroelastosis. An overgrowth of elastic and fibrous fibers in the inner lining of the left atrium and ventricle of the heart. Leads to heart failure early in life.
	Factor IX deficiency (hemophilia B). A sex-linked (females) bleeding disorder characterized by failure of normal blood clotting.
	Hip dysplasia. A deformity of the hip joint, causing pain and leading to lameness.
	Hydrocephalus. Accumulation of excess fluid in the brain and spinal cord, causing an enlarged head.
	Hypotrichosis. A defect of the hair follicles leading to complete hair loss at 6 months of age.
	Idiopathic megaesophagus. A disorder causing enlargement of the esophagus and leading to regurgitation of food and weight loss.
	*Kinked tail.**
	Lysosomal storage diseases. Brain disorders caused by an inheritable deficiency of key enzymes.
	Mucopolysaccharidosis. An inherited enzyme deficiency causing lesions in the bones, brain, and eyes.
	Patent ductus arteriosus. A condition in which a fetal blood vessel does not close at birth, causing a heart murmur and leading to heart failure.
	Porphyria. An accumulation of blood pigments caused by an enzyme defect and causing discoloration in teeth and brownish urine, which turns red under fluorescent light.
	Pyloric stenosis. A narrowing of the muscular outlet of the stomach, causing frequent vomiting, distension of the stomach, weight loss, and cramping. May be corrected surgically.
	*Retinal degeneration.*** Degeneration of the retina at the back of the eye, leading to blindness.

*Common defect, but not a serious problem.

**Prospective owners should screen parents and previous litters.

Breed/Color	Defects and/or Disorders
	Spina bifida. A defective fusion of spinal vertebrae, causing paralysis.
	*Spontaneous nystagmus.** Rapid, involuntary eye movements.
	X-linked muscular dystrophy. Causes a stiff gait ("bunny hop"). Appears at 6–9 weeks of age.
Somali	*Myasthenia gravis*. A disease that causes muscle weakness, including an inability to blink both eyes, breathing difficulty, and regurgitation.
Sphinx	*Alopecia universalis*. Lack of hair coverage.
	Hypotrichosis. A defect of the hair follicles leading to complete hair loss at 6 months of age.
Tricolor cats	*Neuroaxonal dystrophy*. A central nervous system disorder that begins at 5–6 weeks.
	XXY syndrome. Sterility in males.
White cats with blue eyes (sometimes other color eyes)	*Deafness.***

*Common defect, but not a serious problem.

**Prospective owners should screen parents and previous litters.

PROSPECTIVE CAT OWNERS SHOULD BE AWARE THAT MANY CATS ARE SUBJECT TO THE FOLLOWING CONGENITAL DEFECTS AND/OR DISORDERS

	Defects and/or Disorders
Body wall	*Diaphragmatic hernias* (peritoneopericardial and pleuroperitoneal). Abdominal contents enter the chest cavity through an abnormal hole in the diaphragm.
	Inguinal hernia. Hernia in the groin.
	Umbilical hernia. Swelling around the umbilicus (navel). May be surgically corrected.
Bones and joints	*Patellar luxation.* A dislocation of the kneecap, causing pain and lameness. Surgery may help.
	*Polydactyly.** Extra toes.
Cardiovascular system	*Mitral valve malformation.* A malformation of the mitral valve of the left side of the heart, leading to heart murmur and eventual heart failure.
	Persistent right aortic arch. A disorder causing constriction of the esophagus by blood vessels in the chest, which causes a kitten to regurgitate solid food. It may be surgically corrected.
	Pulmonic stenosis. Narrowing or obstruction of the artery leading from the right ventricle of the heart to the pulmonary artery. May produce heart failure.
	Tetralogy of Fallot. A very serious combination of four heart defects leading to poor oxygenation and early death.
	Tricuspid valve dysplasia. A malformation of the tricuspid valve of the right side of the heart. Leads to heart murmur and heart failure.
	Ventricular septal defect. A hole in the wall (septum) between the left and right ventricles of the heart, producing a heart murmur and possible heart failure.

*Common, but not a serious problem.

	Defects and/or Disorders
Digestive system	*Anorectal defects*. Obstruction or stricture of the anus and/or rectum.
Endocrine and metabolic systems	*Diabetes insipidus*. A metabolic disorder due to deficiency of a pituitary hormone, characterized by intense thirst (polydipsia) and large volumes of diluted urine (polyuria).
	Diabetes mellitus. May surface in the first 6 months of life. Characterized by high blood sugar, excessive thirst (polydipsia), and urination (polyuria).
	Neonatal hypoglycemia. Low blood sugar occurring during nursing age. Causes mental confusion, weakness, seizures, and/or coma.
Eyes	*Districhiasis*. An extra row of eyelashes of upper, lower, or both eyelids.
	Divergent strabismus. Wandering (unfocused) eyes, which usually become focused by 3 months of age.
	Microphthalmos. Failure of eye globe to grow to normal size. May lead to blindness.
Hematopoietic and lymphatic systems	*Anasarca*. Swelling of legs and body due to fluid retention.
	Factor VIII deficiency (hemophilia A). A bleeding disorder characterized by failure of normal blood clotting.
	Factor XII deficiency. Mild blood clotting disorder, usually not associated with abnormal bleeding.
	Thrombopathia. A blood platelet disorder causing nosebleeds, bleeding gums, and subcutaneous bruising.
Liver	*Hepatic cysts*. Cysts on the liver that may lead to jaundice or other liver problems.
	Portosystemic venous shunts. Abnormal blood vessel in the abdomen carries blood around, rather than through, the liver. Results in a buildup of toxins, which cause poor growth, salivation, seizures, and death. Surgery can help.
Nervous system	*Cerebellar hypoplasia*. Underdevelopment of the back part of the brain, characterized by lack of balance. Often brought on by feline panleukopenia virus infection in utero or shortly after birth.
Reproductive system	*Cryptorchidism*. Neither, or only one, testicle descends.

Defects and/or Disorders	
	Hypospadias. Abnormal location of male urinary orifice, often on the underside of the penis. May be surgically corrected.
	Os penis deformity. An inability to retract the penis into its sheath. May cause infection and damage.
	Ovarian agenesis. Absence of one or both ovaries.
	Ovarian hypoplasia. The abnormal development of one or both ovaries, resulting in sterility.
	Prepuce anomaly. An abnormal shortening of the penile sheath (foreskin).
	Pseudohermaphroditism. Occurs in both females and males—the external genitalia do not match their actual gender.
	Testicular hypoplasia. The abnormal development of one or both testes, resulting in sterility.
	Triple-X syndrome. Females have 3 X chromosomes instead of 2, preventing normal cycling.
	True hermaphrodite chimeras. Kittens that look like females, born with both ovarian and testicular tissues.
	XO syndrome. Females that do not cycle.
	XX/XY chimeras with testes. Males that have no external testes or scrotum.
Respiratory system	*Tracheal collapse.* Collapsed windpipe, causing coughing and breathing difficulty.
Urinary system	*Agenesis or absence of kidneys.* A fatal disorder if bilateral, caused by abnormal kidney development. If one kidney is affected there may be no sign of a problem.
	Ectopic ureter. A misplacement of the tube or tubes leading from the kidneys to the bladder. Females, especially, are often incontinent.
	Pelvic bladder. Malposition of the urinary bladder. May cause incontinence.
	Urachal anomalies. Cause urine to leak from the navel (umbilicus). Surgery will help.
	Urethral anomalies. Malformations of the tube that takes urine from the bladder outside the body, usually causing frequent urination or incontinence.

Glossary:

Veterinary Medical Terms

and Feline

Diseases/Disorders

Mentioned in the Text

abdominal: Pertaining to the "belly" cavity, containing the stomach, intestines, liver, kidneys, urinary bladder, uterus, etc.

abscess: A collection of pus, usually surrounded by inflamed, damaged tissue.

acquired disease/disorder: A condition that develops after birth, as opposed to one that is present at birth (congenital).

acute: Of sudden or rapid onset, as opposed to chronic.

agenesis: Absence of an organ at birth.

alopecia: Hair loss.

analgesia: Loss of sensation of pain.

anasarca: Fluid in limbs or under the skin. Also called edema.

anemia: Low red-blood-cell count. Often caused by bleeding or chronic kidney disease. Also caused by immune-mediated diseases that destroy red blood cells (hemolytic anemia), or because bone marrow is not producing red blood cells (aplastic anemia).

anomaly: Deviation from the norm, usually congenital.

anorectic: Having anorexia.

anorexia: Loss of appetite.

antibody: A protein the body will manufacture in response to a disease organism or to a vaccine. It helps fight off the disease in the future.

arthritis: Joint inflammation

arthro-: Pertaining to joints.

ascites: An accumulation of fluid in the abdominal cavity, causing abdominal swelling.

aseptic: Free of disease organisms.

atrophy: Wasting away of an organ or tissue.

aural: Pertaining to the ear.

autoimmune disease: A disease in which the body destroys its own tissues.

benign: A tumor or growth that is not malignant (cancerous).

bilateral: Occurring on both sides.

biopsy: Removal of small piece of tissue for microscopic examination.

brachycephalic breeds: Cats with short, pushed-in noses and protuberant eyes.

carcinoma: A cancer that arises in the tissue that lines the skin and internal organs (epithelium).

cardio-: Pertaining to the heart.

castration: Neutering of a male cat by surgical removal of the testicles.

CAT (CT) scan (computerized axial tomography; computed tomography): A specialized imaging technique using X rays. A diagnostic procedure.

cataract: Opacity of the eye lens.

catheter: Tube for insertion into a narrow opening to introduce or remove fluids.

chronic: An ongoing or recurring condition, as opposed to acute.

chylothorax: Accumulation of milky fluid in the chest cavity.

clinical signs: Signs that are able to be seen.

congenital: A condition/disease/defect present at birth, which may surface later in life. Often congenital defects are inheritable, but some are not.

conjunctivitis: Inflammation of the mucous membranes (conjunctival tissue) that line the eyes and eyelids.

cornea: Clear outer-eye covering.

crepuscular: Active at twilight and before sunrise.

Cushing's syndrome: Rare in cats. An endocrine disease causing lethargy, enlarged abdomen, symmetrical hair loss, and thin, easily bruised or torn skin. May lead to diabetes mellitus. Blood tests are used for diagnosis. Medication is not very effective in cats. Surgery to remove affected adrenal gland(s) is often successful.

cutaneous: Related to the skin.

cyanosis: Bluish/purplish discoloration of skin and mucous membranes, due to lack of oxygen in the blood.

cyst: A fluid-filled sac.

dehydration: A lack of water in body tissues. Symptoms include thirst, weakness, nausea, and skin with decreased elasticity.

dementia: Mental deterioration. Lack of normal "thinking."

dermatology: The study of diseases of the skin.

diabetes insipidus: Rare metabolic disorder due to a deficiency of a pituitary hormone, characterized by polydipsia and polyuria.

diabetes mellitus: High blood sugar due to insufficient production of insulin by the pancreas, or lack of insulin absorption by tissues/organs. Symptoms include increased thirst and urination, and weight loss.

dysplasia: An abnormal development of tissue or bone.

dyspnea: Difficult breathing.

dystocia: Difficult birth.

edema: Excessive accumulation of fluid in body tissue, causing swelling.

electrolytes: Ions, such as sodium and potassium, in the blood.

embolus: Blood clot formed in one location that lodges elsewhere.

encephalitis: Inflammation of the brain.

encephalo-: Pertaining to the brain.

endocrinology: The study of the endocrine glands and the hormones they secrete.

enteritis: Intestinal inflammation.

entero-: Pertaining to the intestines.

eosinophilic granuloma complex: A disease of unknown origin (possibly allergic) origin, causing lesions on lips, face, and mouth.

eosinophilic plaques: Raised lesions on mouth or skin, primarily abdomen and thighs.

estrous cycle: Regularly occurring heat cycle.

estrus: The actual heat period.

FeLV: Feline leukemia virus.

FIP (FIPV): Feline infectious peritonitis virus.

FIV: Feline immunodeficiency virus.

FLUTD: Formerly called FUS (feline urologic syndrome). Feline lower-urinary-tract disease.

FUS: See **FLUTD.**

gastro-: Pertaining to the stomach.

gingivitis: Inflamed, swollen, bleeding gums.

hematoma: A blood-filled swelling.

hemobartonella: Blood parasite that can cause hemolytic anemia.

hemolytic anemia: See anemia.

hepato-: Pertaining to the liver.

hereditary: A disease or disorder present at birth that can be traced back to ancestors. May surface later in life.

hydration: Balance of water in the body.

hydrothorax: Fluid around the lungs. May be blood (hemothorax), water (pleural effusion), pus (pyothorax), or chyle (chylothorax).

hyper-: An overproduction, as in hyperthyroidism.

hypercalcemia: High blood-calcium concentration.

hyperplasia: Enlargement.

hyperthyroidism: Normally caused in cats by benign thyroid tumors. Fairly common in old cats. Usually manifested by increased appetite and weight loss.

hypo-: A deficiency or underproduction, as in hypothyroidism.

hypoxia: A deficiency of oxygen in the tissues.

IBD (inflammatory bowel disease): Inflammation of the mucous membranes of the intestines, attributable to many causes. Symptoms include diarrhea, vomiting, and weight loss. Treatment consists of dietary management and some medications.

idiopathic: Of unknown cause.

immune-mediated disease: Disease caused by inappropriate overreaction of immune system.

incubation period: Time between exposure to a disease and the onset of symptoms.

interdigital: Between the toes.

intra-: Within.

-itis: Inflammation of, as in hepatitis (inflammation of the liver).

jaundice: Yellow skin and mucous membranes, usually due to liver disease.

larynx: Opening of the trachea at the back of the throat.

lesion: Disease, or damage-induced tissue abnormality.

lipoma: Fatty, benign tumor.

lymphoma (lymphosarcoma): Cancer of the lymph nodes.

MRI (magnetic resonance imaging): A diagnostic imaging procedure using magnets instead of X rays.

malabsorption: A condition in which the absorption of substances (vitamins and amino acids, for example) in the small intestine is reduced.

malignancy/malignant: Descriptions of a cancer that can spread (metastasize) in the body.

mastitis: Inflammation of the breast.

metastasize: Spread to other parts of the body.

metr-: Pertaining to the uterus.

mucoid: Mucuslike.

mycosis: Disease caused by fungus.

myo-: Pertaining to the muscles.

myositis: Muscle inflammation.

necrosis: Cell death.

neoplasia: Abnormal cell growth.

nephro-: Pertaining to the kidneys.

neuro-: Pertaining to the nervous system.

neurology: The study of the nervous system.

nocturnal: Active at night.

obstipation (megacolon): Obstruction of the colon with feces.

ocular: Pertaining to the eye.

-ology: The study of.

oncology: The study of tumors.

-opathy: Disease or malfunction of.

ophthalmo-: Pertaining to the eye.

oral: Pertaining to the mouth.

orthopedics: The study of bones and joints.

-otic; oto-: Pertaining to the ear.

overiohysterectomy (OHE, "spay"): Neutering of a female cat by surgical removal of the ovaries and uterus.

pancreat-: Pertaining to the pancreas.

perianal: Near or around the anus.

peritonitis: Inflammation of membranes lining the abdominal cavity.

pharynx: Back of the throat leading to the esophagus.

pica: Eating of unnatural or harmful substances (e.g., wool).

pneumo-; pulmono-: Pertaining to the lungs.

pneumothorax: Air in the chest cavity causing lungs to collapse.

poly-: Excessive.

polycythemia: Excessive number of red blood cells.

polydipsia: Increased, excessive thirst.

polyuria: Increased, excessive urination.

pruritus: Itching.

psychogenic: Having an origin in the mind, behavioral.

pulmonary: Related to the lungs.

pupil: Circular opening in the center of the iris, through which light enters the eye lens.

purulent: Containing pus.

pyo-: Pus in, as in pyometra.

pyothorax: Accumulation of pus in the chest cavity.

queen: Female cat that has kittens.

renal: Relating to the kidneys.

rodent ulcer: See **eosinophilic granuloma.**

sarcoma: Malignant tumor of body tissue cells.

shock: See Box, p. 55.

squamous cell carcinoma: Malignant skin tumor in squamous cell (outermost) layer of the skin.

stenosis: Narrowing, as of the spinal canal.

thoracic: Pertaining to the chest cavity.

thrombosis: Condition caused by blood clots.

thrombus: A blood clot.

tomcat: An unneutered adult male cat.

toxic: Poisonous.

trachea (windpipe): Tube that connects the mouth to the bronchi, which branch to the lungs.

trauma: A sudden physical injury.

URI: Upper respiratory infection.

ultrasound: Study of body's interior using sound waves. A diagnostic procedure.

unilateral: Occurring on one side.

uremia: Buildup of poisons in the bloodstream due to kidney failure.

urethra: Tube that carries urine out of the body from the bladder.

vascular: Pertaining to blood vessels.

vertebrae: One of the bones of the spine and tail.

vestibular: Pertaining to the organ of balance, which is controlled by the inner ear and brain.

vulva: Female external genitalia.

Telephone Numbers and Addresses

American Animal Hospital Association (AAHA)

Veterinary hospital referral: call 800-252-2242. Write: AAHA, PO Box 150899, Denver, CO 80215; or e-mail: www.healthypet.com. *Important:* include the zip code of the area in which you need to find a hospital.

ASPCA National Animal Poison Control Center

800-548-2423; $30 consultation fee, payable by credit card. Open 24 hours, every day.

National Pesticide Telecommunications Network (NPTN)

800-858-7378. Free nonemergency information about pesticides, lawn-care and gardening products. Open from 6:30 A.M. to 4:30 P.M. Pacific time, seven days a week, excluding holidays.

Index

I

N
D
E
X

About the Authors

Michael S. Garvey, D.V.M., is a diplomate, American College of Veterinary Internal Medicine (Internal Medicine), and diplomate, American College of Veterinary and Critical Care. He is director of the Elmer and Mamdouha Bobst Hospital at New York's prestigious Animal Medical Center, where he is also chairman of the Department of Emergency Medicine and Critical Care, and staff internist and criticalist. He frequently appears on radio and TV to discuss pet care.

Ann E. Hohenhaus, D.V.M., is a diplomate, American College of Veterinary Internal Medicine (Internal Medicine and Oncology). She is chairman of the Department of Medicine, head of the Donaldson-Atwood Cancer Clinic, and staff oncologist and internist at the Elmer and Mamdouha Bobst Hospital.

Katherine A. Houpt, V.M.D., Ph.D., is a diplomate, American College of Veterinary Behaviorists. She is professor of veterinary physiology and the director of the Behavior Clinic, College of Veterinary Medicine, Cornell University.

John E. Pinckney, D.V.M., has been a director of the Miller-Clark Animal Hospital since 1976. The AAHA-affiliated hospital is one of the oldest exclusively small-animal practices in New York State and has been at its present site since 1903.

Melissa S. Wallace, D.V.M., is a diplomate, American College of Veterinary Internal Medicine (Internal Medicine). She is associate director, head of Renal Medicine Service, and staff internist at the Elmer and Mamdouha Bobst Hospital.

Elizabeth Randolph was for many years a pet-care columnist for *Family Circle* magazine. She is the author of ten pet books, including *How to Be Your Cat's Best Friend, How to Help Your Puppy Grow Up to Be a Wonderful Dog,* and *Dog Training by Bash.* She has also appeared on radio and TV talk shows to discuss pet-care topics.